Intragastric Balloon for Weight Management

Manoel Galvao Neto
Lyz Bezerra Silva
Eduardo N. Usuy Jr.
Josemberg M. Campos
Editors

Intragastric Balloon for Weight Management

A Practical Guide

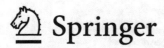

Editors
Manoel Galvao Neto
Department Digestive Surgery
ABC Faculty of Medicine
São Paulo
SP
Brazil

Department of Bariatric Endoscopy
Endovitta Institute
São Paulo
SP
Brazil

Eduardo N. Usuy Jr.
Department of Gastroenterology
and Bariatric Endoscopy
Gástrica Clinic
Florianópolis
Santa Catarina
Brazil

Lyz Bezerra Silva
Department of Surgery
Federal University of Pernambuco
Recife
Pernambuco
Brazil

Josemberg M. Campos
Department of Surgery
Federal University of Pernambuco
Recife
Pernambuco
Brazil

ISBN 978-3-030-27899-1   ISBN 978-3-030-27897-7   (eBook)
https://doi.org/10.1007/978-3-030-27897-7

This Springer imprint is published by the registered company Springer Nature Switzerland AG
The registered company address is: Gewerbestrasse 11, 6330 Cham, Switzerland

Foreword

Obesity has been present throughout human history. Many early depictions of the human body in art and sculpture appear as obese figures. However, it was not until the twentieth century that the World Health Organization became aware that it was the main cause of numerous diseases. It was formally recognized as a global epidemic in 1997. Since then, obesity has become both a major global health subject and issue. Because of its downgrading effects on labor capacity of a great mass of productive adults and restraining their quality of life, the development of more therapeutic options are always welcome and necessary.

It is well established that lifestyle changes as exercises, improvement in nutritional quality intake, and diminishing stress factors are some of the keystones to achieve success in losing weight. Adjuvant drug therapy, with amphetamines, in the past has shown excellent results but severe side effects. Nowadays, the pharmacological therapy for obesity has found its way but still presents a large number of patients with weight regain in a short period of time or nonresponders. Patients who do not achieve the expected results abandon their treatment earlier than the recommended without the acknowledgment of the physician involved in the planned therapy. Nonadherence to medical treatment has been a great challenge.

Due to the necessity of a new approach that could enhance the medical therapy offered until the early 1980s, the first FDA approved model of intragastric balloon, Garren-Edwards Gastric Bubble, was launched. Unfortunately, at that time little was known about obesity, materials that could be applied inside the stomach, and its capacity to adapt to foreign bodies. Many complications as hemorrhagic ulcers and gastric perforation were published. These complications, coupled with disappointing weight loss, led to its discontinuation. The FDA did not approve use of another intragastric balloon in the United States until 2015.

My personal experience with the intragastric balloon started back in 1999 when I had the opportunity to see the new model of the intragastric balloon in Brazil. At that time, the device was seen with skepticism and suspicion. I was a young surgeon and endoscopist, just starting in the bariatric surgery world, and already had contact with a large number of patients that did not fit the indications of bariatric surgery and had already gone through a plethora of known medical treatments. Adding to this population there were super-obese patients that were already benefiting from preoperative weight-loss, lowering surgical complications.

So I went to Italy to meet Professor Santo Bressani Doldi, from the University of Milan, one of the authorities in laparoscopic adjustable gastric bands and intragastric balloons. At that time the balloon was proposed as a test to see if patients would adapt to the lap-band as a bridge between surgery and super-obese patients. Ever since, the method has spread all around the world, not only for super-obese patients but also for patients with lower BMI that do not fit the requirements for surgery.

In 2000, I started the Brazilian multicenter study for the intragastric liquid filled balloon with José Afonso Sallet and Dyker Santos Paiva and participated 16 years later in the Brazilian Intragastric Balloon Consensus, where over 40,000 balloons were reported by 37 different specialists. Both published in 2004 and 2019, respectively.

For the past years the knowledge on obesity, new drug therapies, and the role of the multidisciplinary team in its treatment associated to the intragastric balloon has amplified the weight loss results and its persistence in a higher number of patients, when compared to sole medical treatment.

The intragastric balloon is nowadays an alternative to bariatric surgery for endoscopy-practicing gastroenterologists for patients that do not want or cannot be submitted to surgery.

A great amount of experience has been accumulated for the last 20 years, over 20,000 papers have been published related to weight loss results, complications, hormonal effects, quality of life, and much more subjects associated to the effects of the intragastric balloon.

Manoel Galvao and Josemberg Campos also make part of the history of intragastric balloons in Brazil. The first time I met them was back in 2005 in a Brazilian Bariatric Surgery Meeting, where I was making a live transmission of an intragastric balloon placement. Manoel approached me telling that he was also working with the device. The passion for new technologies in endoscopic approach toward obesity and bariatric surgery back then by Manoel Galvao and Josemberg Campos raised them to the top of the list of the best bariatric endoscopists worldwide. Many have been taught and trained by them globally not only on intragastric balloons but anything related to endoscopic treatment of bariatric surgery complications and endoscopic primary treatment of obesity. Lyz Bezerra and Eduardo Usuy Jr. represent the new generation of bariatric endoscopists, proactive, always seeking for new challenges, "thinking outside the box." No doubt that they already are important leaders in a selective group of young endoscopists, worldwide inside the community of bariatric endoscopy.

This manual compiles all the globally achieved experiences. Many different models of intragastric balloons like gas filled, liquid filled, double balloons, and others have been proposed and are discussed in this wonderful book. Technical approach in placing the balloon is well detailed and can really help newbies. How to manage early and late complications related to the device is masterfully discussed. Last but not least, the role of the dietician, psychological approach, and exercise as the adjuvant treatment is objectively dissected.

I am sure you will enjoy this manual as I have and use it on a daily basis for your clinical practice in leading a multidisciplinary team with the intragastric balloon as your drive to help the obese patient.

Caetano Marchesini, MD
Former President of the Brazilian Society for Bariatric and Metabolic Surgery
Affiliated Professor of the Department of Endoscopy
of Mario Covas Medical School
Member of the Brazilian College of Surgeons
Member at Large LATAM for IFSO
International Member of ASMBS
Curitiba, Brazil

Preface

Intragastric balloon is the oldest endobariatric therapy for obesity with around 20 years on clinical practice that was the starter of the bariatric endoscopy field.

Bariatric endoscopy is a neologism meaning a new term created to define the interface of advanced therapeutic endoscopy with bariatric surgery. Mainly, its interface deals with treating bariatric surgery complications and primary obesity itself even revising secondary obesity (post-operative poor weight loss or weight regain). The interest in bariatric endoscopy among bariatric surgeons, bariatricians, gastroenterologists, and endoscopists is growing fast.

The intragastric balloon has helped thousands of patients in losing weight, improving comorbidities, as a bridge to bariatric surgery, and mostly filling the gap between obesity clinical management, drugs, and the bariatric surgery. Despite the fact that evidence-based scientific information regarding intragastric balloons are abundant and robust on the literature, it is mainly in the form of studies, with a decade of gap since the last textbook about intragastric balloons was published, and since then so many more devices were developed and its use became widespread at the point it has reached the USA (the last country that approved it in 2015 by FDA).

In this publication, the reader will find handy information on how the device has been used all over the world with a practical approach on the various types of devices, its indications, technique, how to recognize and treat complications, and how it fits on clinical practice in a multidisciplinary team environment.

The authors are world leaders in bariatric endoscopy and have worked to provide the reader with a practical and immersive experience in the field of this long-lasting technology that helps battle the world obesity epidemic.

São Paulo, São Paulo, Brazil   Manoel Galvao Neto

Contents

Contributors

Jaber Al-Ali Kuwait Health Sciences Centre, Department of Surgery, Jabriya, Kuwait

Artagnan Menezes Barbosa de Amorim Department of Endoscopy, 9 de Julho Hospital, São Paulo, SP, Brazil

Dilhana S. Badurdeen Division of Gastroenterology and Hepatology, The Johns Hopkins Medical Institutions, Baltimore, MA, USA

Sérgio Alexandre Barrichelo Júnior Department of Bariatric Endoscopy, Healthme Clinic, São Paulo, SP, Brazil

Vitor Ottoboni Brunaldi Endoscopy Unit of the Department of Gastroenterology (Hospital das Clínicas da Faculdade de Medicina da Universidade de São Paulo), University of São Paulo (Universidade de São Paulo), São Paulo, SP, Brazil

Josemberg M. Campos Department of Surgery, Federal University of Pernambuco, Recife, PE, Brazil

Sonja Chiappetta Department of Obesity and Metabolic Surgery, Ospedale Evangelico Betania, Naples, Italy

Ricardo Anuar Dib Department of Endoscopy, Ipiranga Hospital, São Paulo, SP, Brazil

Victor Ramos Mussa Dib Department of Surgery, Victor Dib Institute, Manaus, AM, Brazil

Christopher DuCoin Department of Surgery, Tulane University, New Orleans, LA, USA

Flávio Hayato Ejima Department of Endoscopy, IHBDF – SES, Brasília, DF, Brazil

Moamena El-Matbouly Department of Surgery, Hamad General Hospital, Doha, Qatar

Marcelo Falcão Department of Surgery, Baiana School of the Medicine and Public Health, Salvador, BA, Brazil

Abe Fingerhut Medical University of Graz, Graz, Austria

Ricardo José Fittipaldi-Fernandez Department of Bariatric Endoscopy, Endogastro Rio Clinic, Rio de Janeiro, RJ, Brazil

Manoel Galvao Neto Department Digestive Surgery, ABC Faculty of Medicine, São Paulo, SP, Brazil

Department of Bariatric Endoscopy, Endovitta Institute, São Paulo, SP, Brazil

Eduardo Grecco Department of Digestive Surgery, ABC Faculty of Medicine, Santo André, SP, Brazil

Anna Carolina Hoff Department of Bariatric Endoscopy, Angioskope SP Endoscopic Center, São Paulo, SP, Brazil

Flávio Heuta Ivano Department of Surgery, Paraná Pontifical Catholic University (PUCPR), Curitiba, PR, Brazil

Muhammad Jawad Department of Bariatric Surgery, Orlando Health Institute, Orlando, FL, USA

Mousa Khoursheed Kuwait Health Sciences Centre, Department of Surgery, Jabriya, Kuwait

Vivek Kumbhari Division of Gastroenterology and Hepatology, The Johns Hopkins Medical Institutions, Baltimore, MA, USA

Marina S. Kurian Department of Surgery, New York University, New York, NY, USA

Ariel Ortiz Lagardere Obesity Control Center, Joint Commission Accredited, SRC, International Center of Excellence in Bariatric and Metabolic Surgery, CSG, Tijuana, Baja California, Mexico

University of Baja California, School of Medicine, Mexicali, Baja California, Mexico

University Ibero-Americana, School of Nursing Baja California, Tijuana, Baja California, Mexico

Obesity Control Center, Tijuana, Baja California, Mexico

João Caetano Dallegrave Marchesini Department of Surgery, Marcelino Champagnat Hospital, Curitiba, PR, Brazil

Former President, Brazilian Society for Bariatric and Metabolic Surgery, São Paulo, SP, Brazil

Department of Endoscopy, Mario Covas Medical School, São Paulo, SP, Brazil

Maria Cristina Martins Gastrointestinal Departament, São Rafael Hospital-, AVENIDA SÁO RAFAEL, Salvador, BA, Brazil

Luiz Henrique Mazzonetto Mestieri Endoscopy Unit, Mestieri Clinic, Salto, SP, Brazil

Rena Moon Department of Bariatric Surgery, Orlando Health Institute, Orlando, FL, USA

Rachel Lynn Moore Moore Metabolics & Tulane University, New Orleans, LA, USA

Marcius Vinicius de Moraes Department of Surgery, Pontifical Catholic University, Goiânia, GO, Brazil

Elaine Moreira Department of Bariatric Endoscopy and Gastroenterology, Endovitta Institute, São Paulo, SP, Brazil

Diogo Turiani Hourneaux de Moura Endoscopy Unit of the Department of Gastroenterology (Hospital das Clínicas da Faculdade de Medicina da Universidade de São Paulo), University of São Paulo (Universidade de São Paulo), São Paulo, SP, Brazil

Eduardo Guimarães Hourneaux de Moura Endoscopy Unit of the Department of Gastroenterology (Hospital das Clínicas da Faculdade de Medicina da Universidade de São Paulo), University of São Paulo (Universidade de São Paulo), São Paulo, SP, Brazil

Gabriel Cairo Nunes Department of Endoscopy, University of São Paulo (USP), São Paulo, SP, Brazil

Joel Fernandez de Oliveira Endoscopy Unit of the Department of Gastroenterology (Hospital das Clínicas da Faculdade de Medicina da Universidade de São Paulo), University of São Paulo (Universidade de São Paulo), São Paulo, SP, Brazil

Jaime Ponce Medical Director of Bariatric Surgery, CHI Memorial Hospital, Chattanooga, TN, USA

Uliana Fernanda Pozzobon Psychology, Curitiba, PR, Brazil

Luiz Gustavo de Quadros Department of Digestive Surgery, ABC Faculty of Medicine, Santo André, SP, Brazil

Flávio Mitidieri Ramos Department of Bariatric Endoscopy, Endodiagnostic, Rio de Janeiro, RJ, Brazil

Enrique Rentería-Palomo Division of General and Endoscopic Surgery, Hospital Dr. Manuel Gea González, Mexico City, Mexico

Aida Monserrat Reséndiz-Barragán Department of Endoscopic Surgery, Minimally Invasive Gastrointestinal and Bariatric Surgery, Hospital Dr. Manuel Gea González, Mexico City, Mexico

Martín Edgardo Rojano-Rodríguez Department of Endoscopic Surgery, Minimally Invasive Gastrointestinal and Bariatric Surgery, Hospital Dr. Manuel Gea González, Mexico City, Mexico

Luz Sujey Romero-Loera Department of Endoscopic Surgery, Minimally Invasive Gastrointestinal and Bariatric Surgery, Hospital Dr. Manuel Gea González, Mexico City, Mexico

Kais Assadullah Rona Department of Bariatric and Minimally Invasive Surgery, Tulane University, New Orleans, LA, USA

Alan Saber Department of Surgery, Newark Beth Israel Medical Center, Newark, NJ, USA

Guadalupe de los Ángeles Salinas-Cornejo Division of Clinical Nutrition, Hospital Dr. Manuel Gea González, Mexico City, Mexico

Jimi Izaques Bifi Scarparo Department of Endoscopy, Ipiranga Hospital and Scarparo Scopia Clinic, São Paulo, SP, Brazil

Joao Antonio Schemberk Jr. Department of Endoscopy and Obesity, Obesogastro Clinic, Curitiba, PR, Brazil

Lyz Bezerra Silva Department of Surgery, Federal University of Pernambuco, Recife, PE, Brazil

Thiago Ferreira de Souza ABC Medical, São Paulo, SP, Brazil

Joseph Sujka Department of Bariatric Surgery, Orlando Health Institute, Orlando, FL, USA

Antonio F. Teixeira Department of Bariatric Surgery, Orlando Health Institute, Orlando, FL, USA

Hélio Tonelli Department of Psychiatry, Caetano Marchesini Clinic and FAE Business School, Curitiba, PR, Brazil

Eduardo N. Usuy Jr. Department of Gastroenterology and Bariatric Endoscopy, Gástrica Clinic, Florianópolis, SC, Brazil

Felipe Matz Vieira Department of Bariatric Endoscopy, Endodiagnostic, Rio de Janeiro, RJ, Brazil

Rudolf A. Weiner Department for Surgery of Obesity and Metabolic Disorders, Sana Klinikum Offenbach, Offenbach am Main, Germany

Sylvia Weiner Department for Bariatric Surgery, Nordwest Hospital, Frankfurt am Main, Germany

Idiberto José Zotarelli Filho Department of Endoscopy, Kaiser Clinic, São José do Rio Preto, São Paulo, Brazil

Natan Zundel Department of Surgery, Florida International University, Miami, FL, USA

Part I
Introductory Issues

Intragastric Balloon History

Dilhana S. Badurdeen, Vivek Kumbhari,
and Natan Zundel

The Rapunzel Syndrome

The concept of weight loss using an intragastric balloon (IGB) originated from the Rapunzel Syndrome – a rare psychiatric condition resulting from trichophagia or ingesting hair. The trichobezoar (hairball) occupies the stomach culminating in diminished appetite, postprandial fullness, and weight loss. This concept was used to fill the stomach with a pseudo bezoar – the intragastric balloon, a unique and innovative supposition to induce weight loss.

Minimally Invasive Philosophy: An Alternative to Surgery

The gastric bypass gained popularity in the 1980s as a restrictive and malabsorptive procedure. Even though this is a superb procedure with significant and sustained weight loss, few qualified for it and fewer underwent the procedure due to the apprehension of 'going under the knife' and fear of complications. Thus, it became imperative for surgeons and gastroenterologists to fill this void with a procedure that was easily accessible and less invasive.

The initial experiment of an IGB was conducted in dogs using a 250 ml polyethylene bottle introduced at laparotomy [1]. Subsequently, free-floating rubber balloons that were easy to insert were explored in humans and seemed to reduce hunger. There were no complications noted in the five obese women who participated in the initial 272-day study. The balloons remained inflated for an average of

D. S. Badurdeen · V. Kumbhari
Division of Gastroenterology and Hepatology, The Johns Hopkins Medical Institutions, Baltimore, MA, USA
e-mail: dbadurd1@jhmi.edu; vkumbha1@jhmi.edu

N. Zundel (✉)
Department of Surgery, Florida International University, Miami, FL, USA

© Springer Nature Switzerland AG 2020
M. Galvao Neto et al. (eds.), *Intragastric Balloon for Weight Management*,
https://doi.org/10.1007/978-3-030-27897-7_1

7–21 days, and though encouraging weight loss was noted during periods of inflation, researchers remained in a quandary as to how to keep the balloons from deflating [2].

Early Development

The Garren–Edwards Bubble made its debut in September 1985, after being approved by the U.S. Food and Drug Administration (FDA), as the first IGB, amidst much speculation as a weight loss measure more drastic than stomach stapling and jaw-wiring [3]. It was designed by gastroenterologists Lloyd R. Garren and his wife Mary L. Garren. The *New York Times* reported that 'severely obese Americans were now swallowing stomach balloons to help them reduce their girth'. The bubble was a novel 3 × 4 cm cylinder constructed with polyurethane and a self-sealing valve (Fig. 1.1).

Following routine endoscopy, the bubble was inserted using an introducer tube and inflated with 200 cc of room air with subsequent release into the fundus of the stomach. The exact mechanism of action was unclear and proposed theories included a placebo effect, mechanical, hormonal, or behavioral modification and neuronal pathways to name a few. It was marketed as a temporary device with removal after 4 months [4]. The initial hysteria resulted in the sale of 20,000 bubbles in less than a year. The reality in that first year of placement, based on a retrospective study by Ulicny KS Jr et al., was a mean weight loss of 10.1 kilograms with five patients developing small bowel obstruction from spontaneous deflation of the balloon. Only 33% required endoscopic removal of the balloon whilst the remainder passed the balloon per rectum [5].

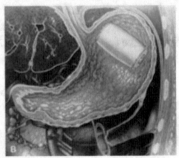

- Approved by FDA In 1985
- Product Details
  - Cylindrical with sharp edges
  - Filled with 200cc of air
  - No removal tool
  - Device not radiopaque
- Product introduction
  - Uncontrolled launch and training
  - Over 20,000 placed in 1st year
  - Poor or no patient follow up program
- Product Performance
  - 3 of 4 studies showed no short-term benefit vs. sham
  - Ulcers / Erosions
  - Deflations (seam, shell and valve failures)
  - Migration /Bowel obstructions
  - Deaths
- Product pulled from the market in 1986

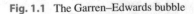

Fig. 1.1 The Garren–Edwards bubble

This was followed by a 24-week double blind crossover study of 90 patients randomized into three groups: bubble-sham, sham-bubble, and bubble-bubble with diet and behavioral modification therapy. Unfortunately, this trial did not demonstrate significantly more weight loss with the gastric balloon compared to diet and behavioral modification alone. Complications included gastric erosions and ulcers, small bowel obstruction, Mallory–Weiss tears, and esophageal laceration [6]. The safety and efficacy were compared to bariatric surgery and demonstrated inferior weight loss [7], resulting in a rather disheartening withdrawal from the market in 1992.

Europe: The Taylor Balloon and the Ballobes Bubble

There was much doubt regarding the efficacy and safety of IGBs, but there were a few that believed the suboptimal weight loss results were a design failure rather than a concept failure and thus the Taylor balloon emerged. In contrast to the Garren–Edwards Bubble, the Taylor balloon was a pear-shaped 550 ml liquid-filled silicone balloon that again remained within the stomach for 4 months. It was filled with normal saline and methylene blue so that the patient would be alerted if there was spontaneous deflation resulting in blue urine. It was introduced in the United Kingdom in 1985. A prospective, multicenter clinical trial conducted at four clinical centers in a total of 60 patients demonstrated an 11.6% decrease in mean total body weight at 16 weeks. Again, seven balloons deflated spontaneously secondary to a manufacturing defect and the design was subsequently modified with no further incidents [8].

The Ballobes bubble was developed in Denmark in 1988. It had a larger volume like the Taylor balloon but was oval in shape. However, in contrast to the Taylor balloon, the 500 ml silicone balloon was filled with air and 10 ml diatrizoate following endoscopy. A randomized double-blind trial of balloon or sham treatment of 3 months' duration did not show a significant difference in weight loss. There were less spontaneous deflations; however, 7% had intolerance secondary to esophagitis [9], likely due to its free-floating nature as it was filled with air (Fig. 1.2).

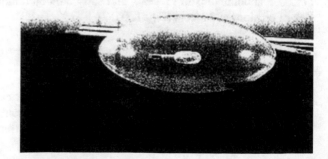

Fig. 1.2 Ballobes intragastric balloon. (Reproduced with permission from - Bariatric surgery, Edited by Nadey S Hakim, Franco Favretti, Gianni Segato and Bruno Dillemans. Copyright @ 2011 Imperial College Press)

Table 1.1 Characteristics of the 'ideal' intragastric balloon

1. Effective
2. Low ulcerogenic and obstructive potential
3. Adjustable volume
4. Soft surface
5. Constructed of durable material
6. Liquid content
7. Radiopaque marker

The Ideal Intragastric Balloon

Following the failure of the IGB in the United States, a comprehensive workshop was held in 1987 to design the ideal IGB. International experts in gastroenterology, surgery, obesity, nutrition, and behavior medicine met in Tarpon Springs, Florida. They developed guidelines for patient selection, insertion, and retrieval techniques and discussed the need for appropriate patient education on nutrition, exercise, and behavior modification [10] (Table 1.1).

In 1991, the BioEnterics® Intragastric Balloon (BioEnterics Corporation) was developed based on the ideal characteristics from the Florida conference. It was a smooth, spherical, 400–700 ml saline- and methylene blue–filled silicone elastomer with a radiopaque filling valve that was introduced endoscopically and remained in the stomach for 6 months. It was initially marketed in Europe, South America, Asia, and Middle East. A randomized controlled trial comparing IGB for 6 months with behavioral modification for 12 months, versus behavioral modification alone showed statistically significant greater weight loss at 6 months in the IGB group (−14.2 vs. −4.8) [11]. Genco A. et al. in his retrospective study of 2515 patients showed not only satisfactory weight loss, but also an improvement in comorbidities, [12] and the feasibility of a first intragastric balloon followed by a second balloon for continued weight loss [13]. Subsequent studies have established the utility of a third and fourth balloon for augmented weight loss over a 6-year follow-up period [14].

The BIB balloon continues to be marketed today as the Orbera® (Apollo Endosurgery, Inc., Austin, TX, USA) balloon. In a multicenter randomized trial of 255 adults with a body mass index of 30–40 kg m^2, Courcoulas A et al. demonstrated a superior weight loss at 3 and 6 months in subjects randomized to IGB with lifestyle intervention compared to lifestyle intervention alone. Due to the larger volume, patients experience more side effects such as nausea (86.9%), vomiting (75.6%), abdominal pain (57.5%), and early balloon removal (18.8%) [15], with a risk of erosions and ulcers (Fig. 1.3).

Gastric Balloons Regain FDA Approval

After a long hiatus, the IGB reappeared on the American market in July 2015, when the ReShape® Duo Integrated Dual Balloon System (ReShape Medical Inc., San Clemente, CA, USA) received FDA approval. It differs from other balloons in

Fig. 1.3 The Orbera®
Intra Gastric Balloon

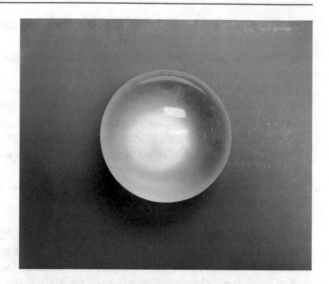

Fig. 1.4 The Reshape®
Duo Integrated dual
balloon system

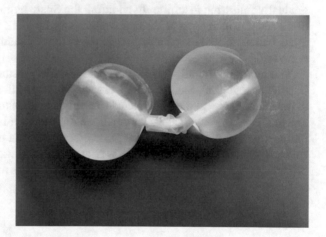

its shape which is thought to conform to the natural curvature of the stomach. It consists of two balloons attached by a flexible silicone shaft to decrease migration into the small bowel in the event of deflation. Each balloon is filled with 450 ml of saline and methylene blue for a maximum capacity of 900 ml. It is placed endoscopically and remains in the stomach for 6 months followed by endoscopic removal. The REDUCE pivotal trial was a prospective, randomized controlled trial of the ReShape IGB. A total of 326 subjects were randomized to IGB with diet and exercise versus sham endoscopy with diet and exercise alone. IGB with diet and exercise had significantly greater %EWL at 24 weeks [16]. The Orbera gained FDA approval in August 2015 (Fig. 1.4).

South America: The Silimed Gastric Balloon (SGB)

The Silimed® gastric balloon (Silimed, Rio de Janeiro, Brazil) is a spherical, 650 ml, silicone-coated balloon with a self-sealing valve like the orbera balloon. It is filled with normal saline, 20 ml Iopamiron contrast, and 10 ml of 2% methylene blue. The balloon is lodged within a sheath that is anchored to the endoscope with a snare and thus introduced using traction. It is easier to place and remove and has superior radiopaque visualization. Mean excess weight loss at 6 months was 11.3 ± 6.2 kg with similar issues of spontaneous deflation and early removal [17].

Adjustable Volume

The Spatz® (Spatz Medical, Great Neck, NY, USA) balloon, though not FDA approved, warrants special mention as the only free-floating balloon with an adjustable volume. This is an important feature that addresses the weight loss plateau seen at 3 months. It also improves tolerance of the IGB as the volume can be increased gradually following insertion. In addition, the Spatz balloon can remain for a total of 12 months increasing additional weight loss by 7–12 kg. The downside to the Spatz balloon is that in order to change the volume an additional endoscopy is warranted (Fig. 1.5).

The adjustable totally implantable intragastric prosthesis (ATIIP)-EndogAst® (Districlass Medical, Saint-Etienne, France) is an air-filled balloon that is attached to the abdominal wall and connected to a subcutaneous totally implantable system and thus overcomes the obstacle of balloon migration. It is placed in a similar fashion as a percutaneous endoscopic gastrostomy tube. In a 1-year multicenter prospective clinical survey mean %EWL at 6 months was 28.7%, however local subcutaneous infection and port erosion have limited its use [18] (Fig. 1.6).

Fig. 1.5 The Spatz® intragastric balloon

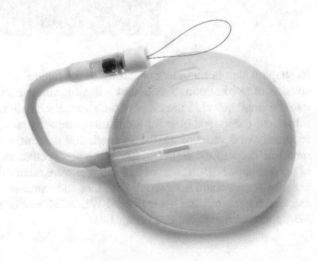

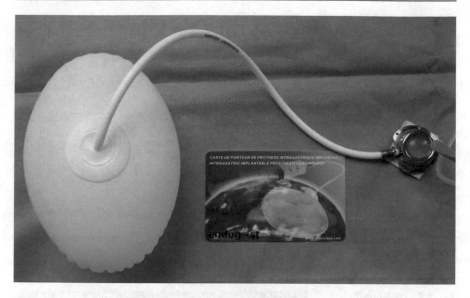

Fig. 1.6   The adjustable totally implantable intragastric prosthesis (ATIIP)-EndogAst®

Is Endoscopy De Rigueur for IGB Placement?

Since a screening endoscopy prior to IGB placement is unlikely to predict the likelihood of complications or intolerance [19], could a balloon be swallowed instead? Indeed, the Obalon® (Obalon Therapeutics Inc., Carlsbad, CA, USA) was the first FDA-approved swallowable balloon developed to circumvent endoscopic placement of the IGB. Endoscopy is expensive and drives up the cost of IGB placement. The Obalon transformed an expensive and time-consuming procedure at a surgical center into a relatively cheaper 10-minute office visit. It is a system of three balloons swallowed 2 weeks apart in the first 3 months of treatment and retrieved with endoscopy 6 months after placement of the first balloon. The 250 cc balloon is deposited in a small capsule that is attached to a 2 *Fr* catheter. Once swallowed, the location is confirmed by X-ray and then inflated with a nitrogen-based proprietary air mixture. The progressive increase in volume to a total of 750 cc over 4 weeks decreases intolerance and early removal secondary to nausea, vomiting, and abdominal pain [20] (Fig. 1.7).

An 'Easy-to-Swallow' Treatment for Weight Loss

The Elipse® (Allurion Technologies Inc., Natick, MA, USA) balloon does not need endoscopy for placement or retrieval. Like the Obalon®, it is swallowed within a capsule and filled with saline during a brief office visit and then months later passes per rectum. It has revolutionized endoscopic IGB placement, to the simplicity of

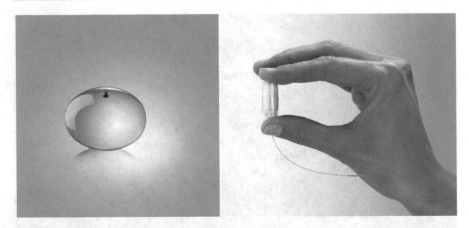

Fig. 1.7 a) The Obalon® Intra Gastric Balloon after inflation b) The capsule containing the Obalon Intragastric Balloon

Fig. 1.8 The Elipse® gastric balloon is folded into a vegetarian capsule and attached to a thin catheter (left). After it is swallowed, the balloon is filled with liquid (right). A US quarter is shown for size comparison purposes

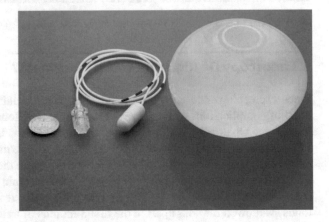

swallowing a pill. It has also eliminated the issue of patients not returning for planned balloon removal [21] (Fig. 1.8).

Balloon-Like Devices: The Semistationary Antral Balloon (SAB) and the Transpyloric Shuttle (TPS)

The semistationary antral balloon is also a pear-shaped saline-filled balloon with a 30 cm silicone duodenal stem for anchorage into the antrum and a 7 g metallic counterweight at the tip. Unlike the Taylor balloon, it is only filled with 150–180 cc saline as the mechanism is believed to be intermittent occlusion of the pyloric opening versus a space-occupying device. In a pilot study of 26 patients, the median weight reduction was 6.5 kg (range 3.7–19.9) at 4 months. Even though the balloon

Fig. 1.9 The Transpyloric Shuttle®

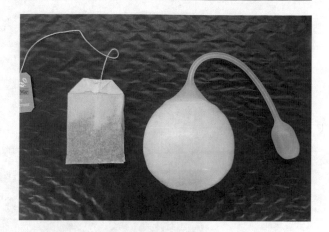

was well tolerated due to its relatively smaller volume distal migration was seen in three patients [21].

The BAROnova Transpyloric Shuttle® (BAROnova, Goleta, CA, USA) is a novel balloon-like weight loss device that is inserted and removed via standard endoscopy. Unlike the conventional balloons, the mechanism of weight loss is delayed gastric emptying. It consists of a large spherical bulb with a mechanical fill connected to a smaller cylindrical bulb by a flexible tether. The larger bulb prevents migration from the stomach, while the cylindrical bulb migrates into the duodenum during peristalsis to enable intermittent obstruction across the pylorus. An initial feasibility study of 20 patients demonstrated 25.1% and 44% excess weight loss at 3 and 6 months, respectively. The ENDObesity II study is a multicenter, randomized, and sham-controlled clinical trial of 270 patients with TPS insertion for 12 months, that demonstrated a mean %TBWL of 9.5% at 12 months (95% C.I. 8.2 to 10.8) in the TPS group compared to 2.8% (95% C.I. 1.1, 4.5) for the Control Group, with an observed difference of 6.7 (95% C.I. 4.5 to 8.8, p < .0001) [22, 23] (Fig. 1.9).

Experimental Devices: Balloon to Butterfly

The butterfly technique is an experimental technique that involves the use of a small butterfly-like, gastric space-occupying device. It consists of an 18-mm × 15-mm, double polyethylene ribbon folded into loops and introduced through an overtube. Upon entry into the stomach, the knot holding the wings together are cut, and the butterfly is released [23].

Comparison of IGBs

Intragastric balloons can be compared based on shape, construction material, volume, filling material, and method of insertion/removal (Table 1.2).

Table 1.2 The comparison of intragastric balloons

	Shape	Material	Volume	Contents	Duration	Method of placement	Method of removal
The Garren-Edwards bubble	Cylindrical	Polyurethane	200 ml	Air	3 months	EGD	EGD
The Taylor balloon	Pear shaped	Silicone	550 ml	Liquid	4 months	EGD	EGD
The Ballobes bubble	Oval	Silicone	500 ml	Air and 10 ml diatrizoate	3 months	EGD	EGD
BIB/Orbera	Spherical	Silicone	400–700 ml	Saline ± methylene blue	6 months	EGD	EGD
Reshape	Bi-lobed	Silicone	450 ml × 2	Liquid	6 months	EGD	EGD
Silimed gastric balloon	Spherical	Silicone	650 ml	Saline, 20 ml Iopamiron contrast and 10 ml of 2% methylene blue	6 months	EGD	EGD
Obalon	Spherical	Silicone	250 ml × 3	Gas mixture	6 months	Swallowed	EGD
Elipse	Spherical	Silicone	550 ml	Saline	4 months	Swallowed	Passed per rectum
Spatz	Spherical	Silicone	700 ml –adjustable	Saline ± methylene blue	12 months	EGD	EGD
Semi stationary antral balloon	Pear shaped	Silicone	150–180 ml	Saline	4 months	EGD	EGD

Conclusion

IGBs earned themselves a credible spot on the armamentarium of short-term weight loss devices and are here to stay. In the future, we anticipate innovative modifications of the IGB that will address side effects such as nausea and gastroesophageal reflux resulting in early removal, technical improvements that will prevent complications including spontaneous deflation, migration, and hyperinflation and solutions for the weight loss plateau seen with current iterations. Balloon placement and removal will be simplified, and duration will progressively lengthen with development of more permanent devices.

However, it is also likely that we will see a shift in gears from space-occupying devices to implantable ones that mimic surgery. Future innovations will be competing with other endoscopic weight loss solutions such as sleeve gastroplasty, and thus will need to be more effective in a shorter duration of time with lasting results. The evolution of the IGB over the last 30 years has been sluggish, to say the least, but has gained momentum in the last few years. This is only a glimpse into the future, which is certain to offer more effective and less invasive solutions than currently available therapy. New device development and research will likely continue until it is possible to deliver custom creations based on subject BMI, comorbidities, weight loss goals, tolerability, and side effect profile. It is unquestionably an exciting time in device development.

References

1. Miller JD. Intragastric prosthesis for management of obesity. World J Surg. 1982;6(4):492–3.
2. Nieben OG, Harboe H. Intragastric balloon as an artificial bezoar for treatment of obesity. Lancet. 1982;1(8265):198–9.
3. Mathus-Vliegen EMH. Is endoscopy really necessary for placing intragastric balloons? Obes Surg. 2018;28(1):169–75.
4. Velchik MG, Kramer FM, Stunkard AJ, Alavi A. Effect of the Garren-Edwards gastric bubble on gastric emptying. J Nucl Med. 1989;30(5):692–6.
5. Ulicny KS, Goldberg SJ, Harper WJ, Korelitz JL, Podore PC, Fegelman RH. Surgical complications of the Garren-Edwards gastric bubble. Surg Gynecol Obstet. 1988;166(6):535–40.
6. Benjamin SB, Maher KA, Cattau EL, Collen MJ, Fleischer DE, Lewis JH, et al. Double-blind controlled trial of the Garren-Edwards gastric bubble: an adjunctive treatment for exogenous obesity. Gastroenterology. 1988;95(3):581–8.
7. Kirby DF, Wade JB, Mills PR, Sugerman HJ, Kellum JM, Zfass AM, et al. A prospective assessment of the Garren-Edwards gastric bubble and bariatric surgery in the treatment of morbid obesity. Am Surg. 1990;56(10):575–80.
8. Marshall JB, Schreiber H, Kolozsi W, Vasudeva R, Bacon BR, McCullough AJ, et al. A prospective, multi-center clinical trial of the Taylor intragastric balloon for the treatment of morbid obesity. Am J Gastroenterol. 1990;85(7):833–7.
9. Mathus-Vliegen EMH, Tytgat GNJ. Intragastric balloon for treatment-resistant obesity: safety, tolerance, and efficacy of 1-year balloon treatment followed by a 1-year balloon-free follow-up. Gastrointest Endosc. 2005;61(1):19–27.
10. Schapiro M, Benjamin S, Blackburn G, Frank B, Heber D, Kozarek R, et al. Obesity and the gastric balloon: a comprehensive workshop. Tarpon Springs, Florida, March 19–21, 1987. Gastrointest Endosc. 1987;33(4):323–7.

11. Fuller NR, Pearson S, Lau NS, Wlodarczyk J, Halstead MB, Tee H-P, et al. An intragastric balloon in the treatment of obese individuals with metabolic syndrome: a randomized controlled study. Obesity (Silver Spring). 2013;21(8):1561–70.

12. Genco A, Bruni T, Doldi SB, Forestieri P, Marino M, Busetto L, et al. BioEnterics intragastric balloon: the Italian experience with 2,515 patients. Obes Surg. 2005;15(8):1161–4.

13. Genco A, Cipriano M, Bacci V, Maselli R, Paone E, Lorenzo M, et al. Intragastric balloon followed by diet vs intragastric balloon followed by another balloon: a prospective study on 100 patients. Obes Surg. 2010;20(11):1496–500.

14. Alfredo G, Roberta M, Massimiliano C, Michele L, Nicola B, Adriano R. Long-term multiple intragastric balloon treatment--a new strategy to treat morbid obese patients refusing surgery: prospective 6-year follow-up study. Surg Obes Relat Dis. 2014;10(2):307–11.

15. Courcoulas A, Abu Dayyeh BK, Eaton L, Robinson J, Woodman G, Fusco M, et al. Intragastric balloon as an adjunct to lifestyle intervention: a randomized controlled trial. Int J Obes. 2017;41(3):427–33.

16. Ponce J, Woodman G, Swain J, Wilson E, English W, Ikramuddin S, et al. The REDUCE pivotal trial: a prospective, randomized controlled pivotal trial of a dual intragastric balloon for the treatment of obesity. Surg Obes Relat Dis. 2015;11(4):874–81.

17. Carvalho GL, Barros CB, Okazaki M, Novaes ML, Albuquerque PC, Almeida NC, et al. An improved intragastric balloon procedure using a new balloon: preliminary analysis of safety and efficiency. Obes Surg. 2009;19(2):237–42.

18. Gaggiotti G, Tack J, Garrido AB, Palau M, Cappelluti G, Di Matteo F. Adjustable totally implantable intragastric prosthesis (ATIIP)-Endogast for treatment of morbid obesity: one-year follow-up of a multicenter prospective clinical survey. Obes Surg. 2007;17(7):949–56.

19. Obalon Balloon System--another gastric balloon for weight loss. Med Lett Drugs Ther. 2017;59(1523):102–3.

20. Al-Subaie S, Khalifa S, Buhaimed W, Al-Rashidi S. A prospective pilot study of the efficacy and safety of Elipse intragastric balloon: a single-center, single-surgeon experience. Int J Surg. 2017;48:16–22.

21. Lopasso FP, Sakai P, Gazi BM, Artifon ELA, Kfouri C, Souza JPB, et al. A pilot study to evaluate the safety, tolerance, and efficacy of a novel stationary antral balloon (SAB) for obesity. J Clin Gastroenterol. 2008;42(1):48–53.

22. Hashiba K, Brasil H, Wada A, et al. Experimental study an alternative endoscopic method for the treatment of obesity: the butterfly technique. Gastrointest Endosc. 2001;53:AB112.

23. Weight Reduction In Patients With Obesity Using The Transpyloric Shuttle®: ENDObesity® II Study, https://2018.obesityweek.com/abstract/weight-reduction-in-patients-with-obesity-using-the-transpyloric-shuttle-endobesity-ii-study/.

Overview of Intragastric Balloons on an Evidence-Based Perspective

Diogo Turiani Hourneaux de Moura,
Joel Fernandez de Oliveira,
and Eduardo Guimarães Hourneaux de Moura

Introduction

Overweight and obesity are a global epidemic and a major public health problem in many countries [1]. It is estimated that in the United States 21% of health-care spending is used to treat obesity-related comorbidities ($ 147 to $ 210 billion per year) [2, 3].

A combination of calorie restriction, regular physical activity, and lifestyle modification associated or not with pharmacotherapy has been used to treat obesity. However, a significant weight loss of 10–15% is rarely achieved or sustained [4]. In contrast, bariatric surgery has the most effective and prolonged response to weight loss [5, 6].

Although bariatric surgery has an excellent outcome in reducing weight and controlling comorbidities associated with obesity, it has a very specific indication and is not risk free [7]. Nevertheless, only 1% of patients who fit the surgical indications are submitted to this type of procedure, due to multifactorial issues (personal preference, financial conditions, and access to information) [8].

There are also some patients with intermediate body mass index (BMI) who do not qualify for bariatric surgery or even who do not wish to undergo such procedure [9]. In these cases, the intragastric balloon (IGB) has become a viable alternative.

The use of IGB has been evaluated in multiple studies, and several concluded that they were effective in promoting short-term weight loss in two-thirds of patients with significant improvements in comorbidities [10].

D. T. H. de Moura (✉) · J. F. de Oliveira · E. G. H. de Moura
Endoscopy Unit of the Department of Gastroenterology (Hospital das Clínicas da Faculdade de Medicina da Universidade de São Paulo), University of São Paulo (Universidade de São Paulo), São Paulo, SP, Brazil

© Springer Nature Switzerland AG 2020
M. Galvao Neto et al. (eds.), *Intragastric Balloon for Weight Management*,
https://doi.org/10.1007/978-3-030-27897-7_2

Types of Balloons

Orbera® (Apollo Endosurgery, Austin, TX, USA) Elastic spherical balloon made from silicone and filled with about 500–700 ml of saline. Inserted and retrieved endoscopically. Used for 6 months. The new device, Apollo 365, can be used for a year (Fig. 2.1).

ReShape Duo® (ReShape Medical Inc., San Clemente, CA, USA) Filled with a saline solution, it is a dual intragastric balloon system, consisting of two balloons attached to each other by a flexible tube. Each balloon has independent channels so that unintentional leaks or deflation in one balloon does not impact the other balloon. Used for 6 months (Fig. 2.2).

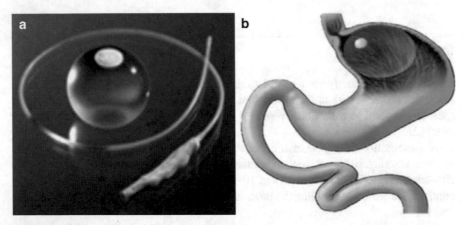

Fig. 2.1 The Orbera® balloon. (NOTE: These pictures are from: [13, 14]). (**a**) Orbera fluid-filled intragastric balloon system. (**b**) Fluid-filled intragastric balloon

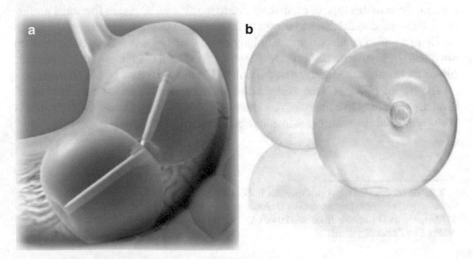

Fig. 2.2 The ReShape Duo® balloon. (NOTE: These pictures are from: [13, 14]). (**a**) Reshape Duo balloon. (**b**) Reshape Duo fluid filled balloon

Spatz® Adjustable Balloon System (Spatz Medical, Great Neck, NY, USA) Saline filled intragastric balloon with an extractable inflation tube for volume adjustment, while the device remains in the stomach. Used for 1 year (Fig. 2.3).

Obalon® Gastric Balloon (Obalon Therapeutics Inc., Carlsbad, CA, USA) Gas-filled balloon with a maximal volume of 250 ml. It is compressed, folded, and fitted in a large gelatin capsule. Once the capsule is ingested, the catheter extends from the stomach to outside the body through the esophagus and the mouth. After balloon inflation, the catheter is detached and removed. One or more balloons can be swallowed during the same session. Used for 12 weeks (Fig. 2.4).

a   b

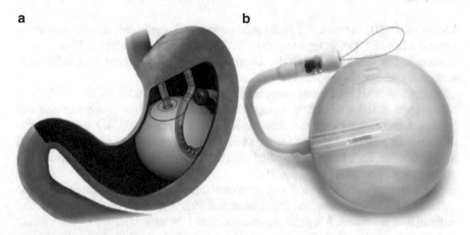

Fig. 2.3 The Spatz® adjustable balloon system. (NOTE: These pictures are from: [13, 14]). (**a**) Adjustable intragastric balloon. (**b**) Spatz adjustable intragastric balloon system

a   b

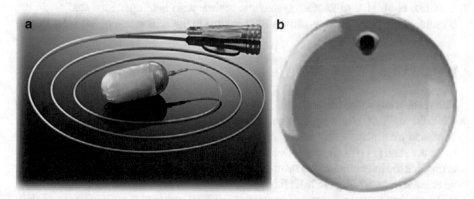

Fig. 2.4 The Obalon® gastric balloon. (NOTE: These pictures are from: [13, 14]). (**a**) Swallowable intragastric balloon system. (**b**) Gas-filled intragastric balloon

Results

The existence of many studies on the subject, often with conflicting results, raises the need for a formal quantitative assessment, such as a systematic review. Systematic review and meta-analysis have become a key practice with the growth of evidence-based medicine, synthesizing a great deal of scientific information, often even contradictory.

Based on this, this chapter demonstrates the results of systematic reviews and meta-analysis of studies evaluating IGB results available in the current literature.

BMI Loss

Moura et al. [10] performed a systematic review and meta-analysis of randomized control trials (RCTs), comparing the effectiveness of intragastric balloon versus sham/diet. For qualitative analysis, 12 studies were selected, and 9 of these were acceptable for quantitative analysis.

Regarding BMI loss, mean percentage reduction achieved with the intragastric balloon was 5.21 kg/m^2 $\pm$ 2.96, compared to 4.1 kg/m^2 $\pm$ 3.62 in the conventional treatment, showing a significant decrease in BMI of 1.1 ($p < 0.050$). A meta-analysis of the results of BMI also demonstrates significant reduction of 2.62 kg/m^2 (95% CI 4.92 to 0.33) in BMI in patients treated with intragastric balloon in comparison with conventional treatment ($p < 0.00001$).

In another systematic review and meta-analysis [11] of 20 RCTs involving 1195 patients, BMI results were analyzed before and after 3 months, of patients with and without IGB treatment. A significant effect size of 1.59 kg/m^2 (95% CI -0.84, 4.03), $p < 0.0001$ was found, in favor of the IGB group. Subgroup analysis revealed an effect size of 2.4 kg/m^2 (95% CI 1.21, 6.1), $p = 0.19$ in the 3-month subgroup (3 studies, 115 patients) and an effect size of 1.34 kg/m^2 (95% CI 0.88, 1.8), $p < 0.0001$ in the >3-month subgroup.

Yorke et al. [12] in another systematic review with heterogeneous studies, in the 6-month duration of therapy, show a BMI change in the IGB group of 5.9 ± 1.0 kg/m^2.

Weight Loss

The meta-analysis of Moura et al. [10] shows a 3.55 kg significant reduction (95% CI -6.20 to -0.90) on weight in patients treated with balloon compared to the conventional treatment.

Saber et al. [11] obtained an effect size of 4.6 kg (95% CI 1.6, 7.61), $p = 0.003$, indicating that the intervention was favored over the control. The subgroup analysis revealed an effect size of 4.77 kg (95% CI 0.51, 9.2), $p = 0.03$ in the 3-month subgroup.

In another systematic review, at the time of IGB removal (medium of 6 months), patients experience statistically significant weight loss ($p < 0.00001$), with a postoperative mean weight loss of 15.7 ± 5.3 kg [12].

The systematic review of Dumonceau et al., including 22 studies with a total of 4,371 patients implanted with the intragastric balloon, showed an average weight loss of 17.6 kg, with extremes of 4.9 and 28.5 kg, with a greater absolute loss in patients with higher initial BMI [13].

% Excess Weight Loss (EWL)

Moura et al. [10] show a mean percentage of excess weight loss in the patients with the intragastric balloon ($n = 238$) of $36.5 \pm 10.8\%$ compared with conventional treatment ($n = 177$) $22.5 \pm 24.2\%$, showing significant increase ($p < 0.05$) in 14.0%.

Ten prospective studies evaluated the IGB outcome after 1 year (6 months after its withdrawal). The percentage of excess weight loss (EWL) ranged from 11% to 51% [14].

Safety

After IGB placement, nausea, vomiting, abdominal pain, eructation, reflux, and dyspepsia are common. These symptoms usually improve after the first week and are usually well controlled with oral medications: proton pump inhibitors, antiemetics, and anticholinergics (scopolamine). Few patients (4–7%) remain very symptomatic after the first 10 days of treatment, and the rate of early withdrawal in studies with Orbera® and ReShape® was 7% and 9%, respectively [14, 15].

Among the patients who need early balloon withdrawal, the most common causes were abdominal pain (17.3%), nausea and vomiting (13.8%), balloon hyper-inflation (12.8%), and intolerance (12%) [12].

Saber *et. al* [11] reviewed the types of complications. Abdominal fullness (6.32 vs. 0.55%, $p = 0.001$), abdominal pain (13.86 vs. 7.2%, $p = 0.0001$), abdominal discomfort (4.37 vs. 0.55%, $p = 0.006$), gastric ulcer (12.5 vs. 1.2%, $p < 0.0001$), nausea (24.79 vs. 11.43%, $p = 0.46$), and flatulence (8.75 vs. 3.89%, $p = 0.0006$) occurred more frequently in the intervention group than in the control group.

Other complications such as small bowel obstruction, grade D esophagitis, gallstone formation, gastroesophageal reflux, hypoxia at IGB removal, cervical esophageal perforation, and pneumonitis after IGB retrieval were not significantly different between the two groups [11].

Comorbidities

Popov et al. [16] performed a systematic review and meta-analysis with 10 RCT and 30 observational studies including 5668 subjects to assess the effect of IGBs on metabolic outcomes associated with obesity.

- Fasting blood glucose (FBG) and glycated hemoglobin A1c (HbA1c): IGB therapy compared with the control groups in RCTs was associated with a reduction in HbA1C of −1.1% (95% CI −1.6, −0.6) and FBG of −12.7 mg/dl (95% CI −21.5, −4) [16]. In a prospective study, the absolute percentage of participants with glycemic levels greater than 100 mg/dl reduced from 50% to 12% [17].
- Low-density lipoproteins (LDL) and triglycerides (TGs): There was no statistical difference between IGB and conventional therapy in RCTs, however TGs decreased by −33.4 mg/dl (95% CI −42, −25) after IGB therapy, 22% reduction from baseline in observational studies. LDL levels decreased as well, but the difference did not reach statistical significance [16]. In the study by Forlano et al. the percentage of patients with hypertriglyceridemia greater than 150 mg/dl reduced from 58% to 19% [17].
- Systolic blood pressure (SBP): There was no difference in SBP between IGB therapy and noninvasive therapy on RCT analysis, −3.4 mm Hg (95% CI −8.5, 1.7), although there was a significant decrease from baseline to final value in the observational analysis of −9.1 mm Hg (95% CI −12, −6.5) [16].
- Liver transaminases: In observational studies both AST and ALT decreased with IGB therapy – ALT, −9 U/l (95% CI −12, −5.2); and AST, −3 U/l (95% CI −5.6, −0.1). The reduction in ALT was 29% from baseline [16].
- Waist circumference: Decreased more after IGB therapy than conventional noninvasive therapy based on RCT analysis – −4.1 cm (95% CI −6.9, −1.4) [16].
- Remission of metabolic conditions: The odds ratio (OR) for diabetes remission after 6 months of IGB therapy was 1.4 (95% CI 1.3, 1.6). The OR for hypertension remission was 2.0 (95% CI 1.8, 2.2); for dyslipidemia remission 1.7 (95% CI 1.2, 2.6) [16].

Final Considerations

Considering the popularity of minimally invasive procedures and the modest effects of nonsurgical treatments such as medications or lifestyle changes, IGB seems well suited to fill that gap, by offering effective weight loss intervention with potentially lower risks, lower costs, and greater patient acceptability. Furthermore, IGB therapy may provide an additional treatment option for patients with metabolic syndrome [14].

Serious complications such as mortality, ulceration, perforation, and balloon migration are rare, making the IGB an acceptable option as a weight-loss intervention, especially in patients with good tolerability to common symptoms after IGB such as nausea, vomiting, and reflux [14].

A recent systematic review and meta-analysis including just RCT proved that IGB therapy in combination with diet was more effective than diet alone for weight loss [10].

The use of Intragastric balloons for obese treatment, in addition to lifestyle modification, is an effective short-term modality for weight loss and improvements in metabolic parameters in selected patients.

References

1. WHO. Global Health. Risks: mortality and burden of disease attributable to selected major risks. Geneva: World Health Organization; 2009. Contract No.: ISBN 978-92-4-156387-1.
2. Finkelstein EA, Trogdon JG, Cohen JW, Dietz W. Annual medical spending attributable to obesity: payer-and service-specific estimates. Health Aff (Millwood). 2009;28(5):w822–31.
3. Cawley J, Meyerhoefer C. The medical care costs of obesity: an instrumental variables approach. J Health Econ. 2012;31(1):219–30.
4. Loveman E, Frampton GK, Shepherd J, Picot J, Cooper K, Bryant J, et al. The clinical effectiveness and cost-effectiveness of long-term weight management schemes for adults: a systematic review. Health Technol Assess. 2011;15(2):1–182.
5. Kumar N, Thompson CC. Endoscopic solutions for weight loss. Curr Opin Gastroenterol. 2011;27(5):407–11.
6. Lee WJ, Lee YC, Ser KH, Chen JC, Chen SC. Improvement of insulin resistance after obesity surgery: a comparison of gastric banding and bypass procedures. Obes Surg. 2008;18(9):1119–25.
7. Flum DR, Dellinger EP. Impact of gastric bypass operation on survival: a population-based analysis. J Am Coll Surg. 2004;199(4):543–51.
8. Buchwald H, Oien DM. Metabolic/bariatric surgery worldwide 2011. Obes Surg. 2013;23(4):427–36.
9. Paulus GF, de Vaan LE, Verdam FJ, Bouvy ND, Ambergen TA, van Heurn LW. Bariatric surgery in morbidly obese adolescents: a systematic review and meta-analysis. Obes Surg. 2015;25(5):860–78.
10. Moura D, Oliveira J, De Moura EG, Bernardo W, Galvao Neto M, Campos J, et al. Effectiveness of intragastric balloon for obesity: a systematic review and meta-analysis based on randomized control trials. Surg Obes Relat Dis. 2016;12(2):420–9.
11. Saber AA, Shoar S, Almadani MW, Zundel N, Alkuwari MJ, Bashah MM, Rosenthal R. Efficacy of first-time intragastric balloon in weight loss: a systematic review and meta-analysis of randomized controlled trials. Obes Surg. 2017;27(2):277–87.
12. Yorke E, Switzer NJ, Reso A, Shi X, de Gara C, Birch D, et al. Intragastric balloon for management of severe obesity: a systematic review. Obes Surg. 2016;26(9):2248–54.
13. Dumonceau JM. Evidence-based review of the bioenterics intragastric balloon for weight loss. Obes Surg. 2008;18(12):1611–7.
14. Force ABET, Committee AT, Abu Dayyeh BK, Edmundowicz SA, Jonnalagadda S, Kumar N, et al. Endoscopic bariatric therapies. Gastrointest Endosc. 2015;81(5):1073–86.
15. Ponce J, Woodman G, Swain J, Wilson E, English W, Ikramuddin S, et al. The REDUCE pivotal trial: a prospective, randomized controlled pivotal trial of a dual intragastric balloon for the treatment of obesity. Surg Obes Relat Dis. 2015;11(4):874–81.
16. Popov VB, Ou A, Schulman AR, Thompson CC. The impact of intragastric balloons on obesity-related co-morbidities: a systematic review and meta-analysis. Am J Gastroenterol. 2017;112(3):429–39.
17. Forlano R, Ippolito AM, Iacobellis A, Merla A, Valvano MR, Niro G, et al. Effect of the BioEnterics intragastric balloon on weight, insulin resistance, and liver steatosis in obese patients. Gastrointest Endosc. 2010;71(6):927–33.

Indications and Uses of the Intragastric Balloon

3

Alan Saber and Moamena El-Matbouly

Introduction

Current therapeutic approaches to obesity are lifestyle changes, pharmacologic treatment, and bariatric surgery. Bariatric surgery has proven to provide the most sustained and effective method for weight loss. However, only 1% of obese patients eligible for the surgical procedure choose to undergo it. The major issues with surgery are difficult access, high costs, patient non-preference, and potential morbidity and mortality [1].

The increased prevalence of obesity has motivated experts in bariatric medicine to advance in minimally invasive endoscopic treatment for obesity management. Abu Dayyeh et al. published a recent meta-analysis proving the efficacy of endoscopic obesity treatment combined with a multidisciplinary treatment plan [2].

The intragastric balloon technique has become an effective method of achieving weight reduction in obese people. The device allows an early feeling of satiety, which is thought to be a consequence of gastric distention. This mechanical intragastric distention during meal time also significantly decreases the amount of food intake [3].

Indications and Contraindications for Gastric Balloon Insertion

Intragastric balloon therapy is an option for obese patients with a body mass index (BMI) equal or greater than 30 kg/m^2 in the United States (US), who have tried and failed previous attempts at weight management with diet and exercise alone, in one of the following situations:

A. Saber (✉)
Department of Surgery, Newark Beth Israel Medical Center, Newark, NJ, USA

M. El-Matbouly
Department of Surgery, Hamad General Hospital, Doha, Qatar

© Springer Nature Switzerland AG 2020
M. Galvao Neto et al. (eds.), *Intragastric Balloon for Weight Management*,
https://doi.org/10.1007/978-3-030-27897-7_3

- For patients with a BMI of 30–35 kg/m^2, intragastric balloon therapy may be used as an early intervention to induce weight loss or to prevent and treat obesity-related medical comorbidities [4].
- For severely obese patients, such as those with a BMI greater than 50 kg/m^2, intragastric balloon therapy may be used as a bridging intervention prior to bariatric surgery. These patients would be at risk of developing anesthesia-related complications during surgery or technical difficulty due to hepatomegaly or increased intra-abdominal fat [5].
- For patients who are eligible to bariatric surgery but refuse it and consider it "too risky," or those who lack access to facilities providing bariatric surgery; intragastric balloon can be used as an alternative method to induce weight loss.

Contraindications of Intragastric Balloon

Both absolute and relative contraindications for intragastric balloon are in Table 3.1.

Uses and Application of Intragastric Balloon in Obese Patients

Body Weight Loss

In comparative studies of the Orbera® balloon (Apollo Endosurgery, Inc., Austin, TX, USA), Giardiello et al. and De Castro et al. indicated that the mean weight loss associated with IGB therapy ranged between 10.5 and 13.7 kg after 3 months, and between 12 and 26.3 kg after 6 months [6, 7].

Additionally, the initial body weight loss (BWL) following intragastric balloon placement was associated with significant long-term weight maintenance as shown in the Dogan et al. study [8]. The percentage of BWL 1 month after intragastric balloon placement was significantly associated with weight loss after 6, 12, and 18 months.

Saber et al. showed in a meta-analysis that BMI loss was 1.59 and 1.34 kg/m^2 for overall and 3 month, respectively; EWL was 14.25 and 11.16% for overall and

Table 3.1 Absolute and relative contraindications for intragastric balloon [5]

Absolute contraindications	Relative contraindications
Previous gastric surgery	Previous abdominal surgery
Coagulation disorders	Large hiatal hernia
Bleeding lesion in the upper gastrointestinal tract	Inflammatory bowel disease
Pregnancy or desire to become pregnant during treatment	Chronic nonsteroidal anti-inflammatory drug (NSAID) use
Alcoholism or drug addiction and severe liver disease	Uncontrolled psychiatric disorders

3 month, respectively; and weight loss was 4.6 and 4.77 kg for overall and 3-month weight loss, respectively [9]. They also showed a significant effect size that favored fluid-filled IGBs over air-filled intragastric balloon [9].

Improvement in Obesity-Related Comorbidities and Metabolic Diseases

Crea et al. assessed 143 obese patients after insertion of Orbera® balloon with 12-months follow-up. They found that the incidence of metabolic syndrome declined from 34.8% (before balloon insertion) to 14.5%, 13%, and 11.6% at the time of removal, at the 6-month follow-up, and at the 1-year follow-up, respectively [10]. Likewise, the occurrence of hyperuricemia, hypertriglyceridemia, and hyper-cholesterolemia decreased from 26.1%, 37.7%, and 33.4% to 25.4%, 14.5%, and 16.7%, respectively. At the time of removal, 25.9%, 15.2%, and 16.7%, respectively, at the 6-month follow-up, and 26.4%, 17.4%, and 18.9%, respectively, at the 1-year follow-up [10].

Similarly, in a large multicenter European study, Genco et al. mentioned that the percentage of patients with comorbidities at baseline and at the 3-year follow-up was 29% and 16% for hypertension, 15% and 10% for diabetes mellitus, 20% and 18% for dyslipidemia, 32% and 21% for hypercholesterolemia, and 25% and 13% for osteoarthropathy, respectively [11].

A randomized controlled study showed that intragastric balloon therapy improved the histology of nonalcoholic steatohepatitis [12].

Alteration in Gastrointestinal Hormones

A study with 40 obese patients who underwent balloon placement indicated no effect on ghrelin levels when patients were fasting or meal-suppressed [13]. In another study, 17 patients with nonmorbid obesity underwent balloon placement, and fasting plasma ghrelin concentrations significantly decreased (3.2–1.9 ng/mL; $P = 0.021$) [14].

Mathus-Vliegen et al. evaluated fasting and postprandial cholecystokinin and pancreatic polypeptide secretion after 13 weeks of balloon treatment in 42 obese patients. Baseline and meal-stimulated cholecystokinin levels were decreased [15].

Conclusion

Intragastric balloon is showing a promise in improving lifestyle and weight loss in obese patients. It offers a minimally invasive and effective method for managing obesity and associated conditions. It can be used as a bridging step for super-obese patients to lose weight and to improve obesity-related comorbidities.

References

1. Buchwald H, Oien DM. Metabolic/bariatric surgery worldwide 2011. Obes Surg. 2013;23:427–36.
2. Abu Dayyeh BK, Kumar N, Edmundowicz SA, Jonnalagadda S, Larsen M, Sullivan S, Thompson CC, Banerjee S. ASGE Bariatric Endoscopy Task Force systematic review and meta-analysis assessing the ASGE PIVI thresholds for adopting endoscopic bariatric therapies. Gastrointest Endosc. 2015;82:425–438.e5.
3. Geliebter A, Melton PM, McCray RS, Gage D, Heymsfield SB, Abiri M, Hashim SA. Clinical trial of silicone-rubber gastric balloon to treat obesity. Int J Obes. 1991;15:259–66.
4. Martins Fernandes FA Jr, Carvalho GL, Lima DL, et al. Intragastric balloon for overweight patients. JSLS. 2016;20(1):e2015.00107.
5. Göttig S, Weiner RA, Daskalakis M. Preoperative weight reduction using the intragastric balloon. Obes Facts. 2009;2(Suppl 1):20–3.
6. Giardiello C, Borrelli A, Silvestri E, Antognozzi V, Iodice G, Lorenzo M. Air-filled vs. water-filled intragastric balloon: a prospective randomized study. Obes Surg. 2012;22:1916–9.
7. De Castro ML, Morales MJ, Del Campo V, Pineda JR, Pena E, Sierra JM, Arbones MJ, Prada IR. Efficacy, safety, and tolerance of two types of intragastric balloons placed in obese subjects: a double-blind comparative study. Obes Surg. 2010;20:1642–6.
8. Dogan UB, Gumurdulu Y, Akin MS, Yalaki S. Five percent weight lost in the first month of intragastric balloon treatment may be a predictor for long-term weight maintenance. Obes Surg. 2013;23:892–6.
9. Saber AA, Shoar S, Almadani MW, Zundel N, Moataz M. Bashah MM, Rosenthal R. Efficacy and safety of first-time single intra-gastric balloon in weight loss: a systematic review and meta-analysis of randomized controlled trials. Obes Surg. 2017 Feb; 27(2):277–287.
10. Crea N, Pata G, Della Casa D, Minelli L, Maifredi G, Di Betta E, Mittempergher F. Improvement of metabolic syndrome following intragastric balloon: 1 year follow-up analysis. Obes Surg. 2009;19:1084–8.
11. Genco A, López-Nava G, Wahlen C, Maselli R, Cipriano M, Sanchez MM, Jacobs C, Lorenzo M. Multi-centre European experience with intragastric balloon in overweight populations: 13 years of experience. Obes Surg. 2013;23:515–21.
12. Lee YM, Low HC, Lim LG, Dan YY, Aung MO, Cheng CL, Wee A, Lim SG, Ho KY. Intragastric balloon significantly improves nonalcoholic fatty liver disease activity score in obese patients with nonalcoholic steatohepatitis: a pilot study. Gastrointest Endosc. 2012;76:756–60.
13. Mathus-Vliegen EM, Eichenberger RI. Fasting and meal-suppressed ghrelin levels before and after intragastric balloons and balloon-induced weight loss. Obes Surg. 2014;24:85–94.
14. Mion F, Napoléon B, Roman S, Malvoisin E, Trepo F, Pujol B, Lefort C, Bory RM. Effects of intragastric balloon on gastric emptying and plasma ghrelin levels in non-morbid obese patients. Obes Surg. 2005;15:510–6.
15. Mathus-Vliegen EM, de Groot GH. Fasting and meal-induced CCK and PP secretion following intragastric balloon treatment for obesity. Obes Surg. 2013;23:622–33.

Brazilian Experience on the Use of Intragastric Balloons

4

Manoel Galvao Neto, Lyz Bezerra Silva, Eduardo N. Usuy Jr., and Josemberg M. Campos

Introduction

A consensus meeting was organized in Brazil, gathering expert endoscopists, with the aim of filling the gap of intragastric balloons (IGB) technique and follow-up standardization. The goal of the meeting was to reach a consensus on best practice based on scientific literature and practice of experts [1].

Prior to the meeting, a questionnaire was sent to all participants to compile data of IGB procedures performed by the group. These data comprised a total of 41,866 IGB cases. In addition to providing a source of information for the meeting, they reflect the panel's extensive experience in this procedure.

Brazilian Experience Data

The total number of IGBs in the group's experience were 41,866 implants and 38,120 explants. Mean patient age was 37.7 years, with 75.9% being female, on average. The mean pre-procedure BMI was 34.4 kg/m^2. The minimum reported

M. Galvao Neto
Department Digestive Surgery, ABC Faculty of Medicine, São Paulo, SP, Brazil

Department of Bariatric Endoscopy, Endovitta Institute, São Paulo, SP, Brazil

L. B. Silva · J. M. Campos
Department of Surgery, Federal University of Pernambuco, Recife, PE, Brazil

E. N. Usuy Jr. (✉)
Department of Gastroenterology and Bariatric Endoscopy, Gástrica Clinic, Florianópolis, SC, Brazil
e-mail: usuy@usuy.com.br

© Springer Nature Switzerland AG 2020
M. Galvao Neto et al. (eds.), *Intragastric Balloon for Weight Management*,
https://doi.org/10.1007/978-3-030-27897-7_4

pre-procedure BMI was 25 kg/m² and the maximum was 102 kg/m² (patient with dwarfism) (Table 4.1).

The most used balloon was the non-adjustable, fluid-filled Orbera® (Apollo Endosurgery Inc., Austin, TX, USA), totaling 32,735 implants (78.2%) (Table 4.2). The mean percentage of total body weight (TBW) loss was 18.4 ± 2.9%. The minimum %TBW loss reported was 0.0% and the maximum was 52%. Patients lost a mean of 18.3 ± 4.4 kg, with a minimum reported TBW loss (kg) of 0 kg and maximum of 87.5 kg. The failure rate (defined as %TBW loss <10%) was 8.3 ± 6.7% (Table 4.3).

The most common adverse events were hyperinflation (0.9%) and spontaneous deflation (0.8%). Migrations needing surgical treatment happened in 24 cases, most common with air-filled balloons (1%). Gastric ulcers occurred in 141 cases, more common with the adjustable balloon (5.7%). There were no esophageal or gastric perforations during the implant procedure and a total of six perforations during the explant, mostly with the Silimed® balloon, a device with a more rigid structure and difficult removal (Table 4.4).

Table 4.1 Demographic data

Variable	Mean ± SD	Minimum	Maximum
Male (%)	24.1 ± 8.6	8.0	45.0
Female (%)	75.9 ± 8.6	55.0	92.0
Minimum age (yrs)	14.3 ± 2.3	10.0	18.0
Maximum age (yrs)	71.2 ± 5.0	62.0	83.0
Mean age (yrs)	37.7 ± 4.4	28.0	45.0
Minimum BMI (kg/m²)	26.8 ± 1.2	25.0	30.0
Maximum BMI (kg/m²)	63.8 ± 12.0	43.0	102.0
Mean BMI (kg/m²)	34.4 ± 2.4	30.0	42.0

Table 4.2 Number of implanted and explanted balloons, by brand

Balloon type	Implants (N)	Explants (N)
Orbera®	32,735	30,394
Medicone®	5172	4429
Silimed®	1882	1788
Spatz®	1020	388
Helioscopie®	1054	1120
Bioflex®	3	0
Others	0	1
Total	41,866	38,120

Table 4.3 Weight loss results from IGB

Variable	Mean ± SD	Minimum	Maximum
TBW (%) mean	18.43 ± 2.92	13.0	25.0
TBW (kg) mean	18.3 ± 4.39	12.50	32.50
BMI reduction (mean)	7.23 ± 3.13	3.50	18.0
Failure (%)	8.33 ± 6.70	0.50	32.0

Table 4.4 Adverse events

	Orbera	Medicone	Silimed	Spatz	Helioscopie	Total
N	32,735	5172	1882	1020	1054	41,866
Hyperinflation[a]	164 (0.5%)	29 (0.56%)	1 (0.05%)	5 (0.49%)	6 (0.57%)	205 (0.49%)
Hyperinflation[b]	146 (0.45%)	4 (0.08%)	12 (0.64%)	4 (0.39%)	0 (0%)	166 (0.40%)
Spontaneous deflation	206 (0.63%)	75 (1.45%)	50 (2.66%)	11 (1.08%)	23 (2.18%)	365 (0.87%)
Migrations[c]	8 (0.02%)	3 (0.06%)	2 (0.11%)	0 (0%)	11 (1.04%)	24 (0.06%)
Migrations[b]	28 (0.09%)	10 (0.19%)	29 (1.54%)	2 (0.20%)	10 (0.95%)	79 (0.19%)
Ulcer[a]	13 (0.04%)	5 (0.1%)	0 (0%)	6 (0.59%)	4 (0.36%)	28 (0.07%)
Ulcer[b]	32 (0.10%)	20 (0.39%)	5 (0.27%)	52 (5.10%)	4 (0.38%)	113 (0.27%)
Bleeding[a]	12 (0.04%)	5 (0.1%)	2 (0.11%)	1 (0.10%)	0 (0%)	20 (0.05%)
Bleeding[b]	30 (0.09%)	2 (0.04%)	5 (0.27%)	2 (0.20%)	0 (0%)	39 (0.09%)
Perforations on implant	0 (0%)	0 (0%)	0 (0%)	0 (0%)	0 (0%)	0 (0%)
Perforations (during treatment)	9 (0.03%)	2 (0.04%)	2 (0.11%)	1 (0.10%)	0 (0%)	14 (0.03%)
Perforations on explant	2 (0.01%)	0 (0%)	4 (0.22%)	0 (0%)	0 (0%)	6 (0.01%)
Total	650 (1.99%)	155 (3.0%)	112 (5.95%)	84 (8.24%)	58 (5.5%)	1059(2.53%)

[a]Treated by balloon removal
[b]Treated conservatively
[c]Treated surgically

Intolerance leading to early removal happened in 2.2% ($n = 928$). The air-filled device had the lowest early removal rate (0.8%), probably because of its lightweight leading to less symptoms. Fungal infection of the device occurred in 5.8% of the cases, more frequent in the air-filled balloon (14.9%), probably because of its double-layer characteristic.

There were 12 deaths (0.03%) reported during the presence of the balloon, with a variety of causes, with balloon-related deaths in only three cases. The balloon-related causes were gastric rupture due to overfeeding in a superobese patient ($n = 1$), pulmonary aspiration with uncoercive vomiting 4 days after implant ($n = 1$), and one case of pulmonary embolism ($n = 1$), which may not have been caused directly by the balloon.

Consensus Results

Indications and Contraindications

Placement

According to the experts, minimum age for balloon implant is 12 years, after established puberty, with multidisciplinary evaluation and parental consent. There is no maximum age limit for implant, each case should be considered individually.

The minimum BMI for balloon implant is 25 kg/m^2, after failure of clinical treatment, with no influence of BMI on choice of balloon type.

Absolute Contraindications
Esophageal, gastric, and duodenal ulcers were considered absolute contraindications for balloon implant, owing to the increased risk of perforation. Previous gastric surgery was considered a contraindication by 93.8% of the participants.

Relative Contraindications
Gastric angioectasias without signs of bleeding (75%), eosinophilic esophagitis (81.3%), immunocompetent HIV positive patient (96.9%), and uncontrolled/untreated psychiatric disorders (75.8%).

Pre-procedure Evaluation and Multidisciplinary Follow-Up

Prior Endoscopy and Exams
Regarding pre-procedure evaluation, prior endoscopy was not considered essential (84.4%), since it is possible to evaluate the stomach during the implant procedure. No imaging exams were considered mandatory before the procedure (84.4%), unless there is clinical indication for such, and/or the request of the anesthesiologist. Regarding laboratory exams, no consensus was reached, 41.9% agree that these should always be requested.

Technique

Balloon Implant
It is recommended that the minimum required structure is an outpatient clinic with advanced life support and patient transfer service available if needed (83.9%).

Anesthesia
No consensus was reached regarding sedation: 14.7% prefer conscious sedation; 41.2% prefer deep/general sedation, without orotracheal intubation or the presence of an anesthesiologist; 17.7% prefer a deep/general sedation without orotracheal intubation, performed by anesthesiologist and 26.5% prefer to have an anesthesiologist choose and perform the sedation.

Balloon Volume
No consensus was reached for recommended maximum balloon filling volume. For the adjustable liquid balloon, 54.8% agree that minimum initial filling volume is between 500 and 600 ml; 38.7% believe minimum volume should be between 400 and 500 ml. At the readjustment session, there was no consensus on the additional filling volume: 42.9% recommend a maximum additional volume of 200–300 ml, 25% recommend 100–200 ml, 14.3% recommend 300–400 ml.

For downward adjustments, owing to intolerance (nausea and vomiting), 59.3% believe the minimum filling volume to remain in the adjustable balloon is between 300 and 400 ml, leading to symptom improvement and subsequent upward adjustment.

Balloon Explant

At least 2 days of liquid diet is recommended prior to balloon removal (90.9%), followed by 12-hour fasting (80.7%). Ingestion of cola carbonated drinks (without sugar) is useful as preparation for balloon removal, since this helps to clean any food residues from the stomach (78.1%).

Anesthesia

Regarding explant sedation, once again no consensus was reached.

Technique

A hybrid jaw grasper (alligator + rat tooth) is the preferred accessory for balloon removal (75%). In selected cases, an esophageal overtube may be used to facilitate removal (74.1%); whilst 56.7% also agree that a small amount of vegetable cooking oil can be selectively used to lubricate the esophagus and 30% believe it should always be used [2].

Post-implant Follow-Up

Medications recommended to be administered during the adaptation period to attenuate symptoms are ondansetron, hyoscine, corticosteroid, proton pump inhibitor (PPI), analgesic and dimenhydrinate, usually for up to 3–5 days after implant. The use of PPIs should be maintained throughout treatment (87.5%). Metoclopramide is not recommended in the adaptation period (70.4%) because it increases gastrointestinal motility and may worsen symptoms. Anti-inflammatory drugs are not recommended (96.3%), due to the risk of gastric injury.

Adverse Events

IGB removal is recommended in cases of moderate or severe pancreatitis (90.6%), gastrointestinal bleeding successfully treated only by endoscopic methods (76.5%), gastric ulcer with nonadjustable balloon (90%), recurrent antral impaction (86.7%), symptomatic hyperinflation (96.9%), and recurrent hydro electrolytic disorder (76.7%). In the case of antral impaction, the balloon can be repositioned. In the event of pregnancy, the balloon should be removed (81.3%), preferably in the second trimester.

In the case of adjustable balloon, 53.9% believe the presence of an ulcer demands balloon removal, even if the patient does not agree. In cases where removal is not performed, repositioning the balloon-filling catheter together with clinical treatment is recommended, except in cases of deep ulcers, with increased risks of perforation, in which case the removal is necessary.

In the presence of mild pancreatitis, removal is not mandatory (76.7%). In the cases of gastrointestinal bleeding that is spontaneously stopped, the balloon can also remain in place (84.4%). In the presence of severe erosive esophagitis, 87.1% recommend that the balloon not be removed before appropriate treatment, due to the increased risk of esophageal lesion during removal. The Mallory–Weiss Syndrome cases should also be treated with the balloon in place.

Conclusions

The full version of the Brazilian Intragastric Balloon Consensus has been published as a scientific paper [1]. This consensus and data collection represents the extensive experience of Brazilian experts, a country that pioneered IGB therapy.

References

1. Neto MG, Silva LB, Grecco E, de Quadros LG, Teixeira A, Souza T, et al. Brazilian Intragastric Balloon Consensus Statement (BIBC): practical guidelines based on experience of over 40,000 cases. Surg Obes Relat Dis. 2018;14(2):151–9.
2. Neto G, Campos J, Ferraz A, Dib R, Ferreira F, Moon R, et al. An alternative approach to intragastric balloon retrieval. Endoscopy. 2016;48(Suppl 1 UCTN):E73.

How the Intragastric Balloon Fits in a Service of Bariatric Endoscopy: Brazilian Perspective

Jimi Izaques Bifi Scarparo and Ricardo Anuar Dib

Introduction

Bariatric endoscopy is a more conservative and less aggressive approach when compared to bariatric surgery. Different options are available, such as the balloon, endoscopy sleeve gastroplasty, gastric drainage, all established in the world and approved in several countries. However, certainly, the intragastric balloon is today, among them, the most used and most accessible.

The intragastric balloon (IGB) is considered a safe technique, with a low rate of complications and mortality, quite easily performed by specialist physicians. Its use has been increasing, because it is a temporary, reversible, and repeatable technique, with a good weight loss rate.

In this chapter, we will discuss the Brazilian perspective for use of IGBs in a bariatric endoscopy service, where more than 40,000 balloons have been implanted in the last 15 years [3],

Brazilian Perspective

A consensus meeting was held in São Paulo, Brazil, in June 2016, bringing together 39 Brazilian endoscopists with extensive experience in IGBs from all regions of the country. Topics on patient selection, indications, contraindications, multidisciplinary follow-up, technique, and adverse events were discussed in the form of

J. I. B. Scarparo (✉)
Department of Endoscopy, Ipiranga Hospital and Scarparo Scopia Clinic,
São Paulo, SP, Brazil
e-mail: drjimi@scarparoscopia.com

R. A. Dib
Department of Endoscopy, Ipiranga Hospital, São Paulo, SP, Brazil

© Springer Nature Switzerland AG 2020
M. Galvao Neto et al. (eds.), *Intragastric Balloon for Weight Management*,
https://doi.org/10.1007/978-3-030-27897-7_5

questions. After electronic voting, a consensus was defined when there was ≥70% agreement [1].

Experts were also requested to provide data on their experience with IGBs. The selected experts discussed and reached a consensus on 76 questions, mainly concerning specific indications and contraindications for the procedure; technical details, such as patient preparation, minimum balloon-filling volume, and techniques for implant and explant; patient follow-up and recommended medication for the adaptation period; and adverse event management.

The overall Brazilian expert data encompassed 41,863 IGBs, with a mean percentage total weight loss of 18.4% ± 2.9%. The adverse event rate after the adaptation period was 2.5%, the most common being hyperinflation (0.9%) and spontaneous deflation (0.8%) of the device. The early removal rate due to intolerance was 2.2%.

The consensus reflects Brazil's significant experience with this device. The experience of over 40,000 cases shows that the device leads to satisfactory weight loss with a low rate of adverse events [1].

One of the issues discussed in this consensus was the minimum BMI required to implant a balloon, in Brazil. There was a consensus that a BMI equal to or greater than 25 Kg/m² would be the minimum required to use the balloon as treatment, since obesity is a progressive and recurrent disease.

Indications for Balloon in a Bariatric Endoscopy Service

BMI Between 25 and 35 Kg/m²

This is the largest population among all of those who are overweight, and the main public for which IGBs are used in Brazil. Usually, this population has already tried and failed the use of medications, exercises, and diets, with a history of successive weight regain. Often, the indication comes from cardiologists to assist in the issues of hypertension associated with obesity, or endocrinologists who have tried drug treatment with little success. In some cases, gynecologists indicate IGBs for improvement in fertility. Orthopedists also indicate IGBs for relief of the musculoskeletal system disorders, such as locomotion difficulty in the elderly. Also, one of the main reasons for seeking treatment in this range of BMI is improvement in aesthetics, for which an average weight loss of 20% is very inviting [1, 4–6].

BMI Between 35 and 40 Kg/m²

For this population, there is an option of choosing between balloon implantation and bariatric surgery. The patient with a BMI between 35 and 40 may not benefit sufficiently from a loss of 20% (IGB) of the total weight. So, a very careful study for the best decision should be done, encompassing not only the comorbidities but also perhaps the psychological profile, personal preferences, and financial situation, among others. In Brazil, bariatric surgery is covered by health insurance for this BMI range, especially in the presence of comorbidities. The intragastric balloon, however, is not covered by health insurances, and sometimes the financial aspect is what helps in the final decision for treatment [5–7].

Super-Obese with a BMI 50 or Higher, to Reduce Surgical Risk Before Bariatric Surgery

This was the first authorized use for IGBs in Brazil, in the late 1990s [8]. Still, there are not enough studies showing the cost–benefit analysis of this approach. This is also the only exception for the possibility of coverage by some health insurances. All the risks involved in performing this procedure in super-obese patients, such as difficult anesthesia, more frequent complications, and lesser chance of success, should be considered. Nevertheless, some specialized services act on this patient with great interest, especially those who have a bariatric surgeon in their clinical body, or where the endoscopist himself or herself is also a bariatric surgeon.

BMI 40 or Higher, Who Do Not Want or Cannot Undergo Bariatric Surgery

It is necessary to consider that there are patients who, despite a precise indication for bariatric surgery, do not want to perform it, either because of the risks involved or because they are not psychologically prepared. There are also patients who have the indication but cannot undergo surgery due to its clinical restrictions where risk does not supplant the benefit. Optionally, the IGB represents a less invasive, temporary device with good results [5, 2].

Final Considerations

The intragastric balloon has assumed an important role in any bariatric endoscopy service. In Brazil, it is mainly used for indications described above, which virtually encompasses any patient who is overweight, with comorbidities or not. The authors believe that the IGB as a medical treatment will still have a lot of growth in the country.

Brazil has one of the largest, if not the largest, casuistics of IGBs in the world [1], and this treatment will still gain more notoriety among physicians who work in obesity as this disease continues to grow and advance as a pandemic. The 20% weight loss achieved can be considered acceptable, with improvement in quality of life and comorbidities. The prejudice against this device will decrease with the large number of recent publications, showing good results in sustainable weight loss and safety.

References

1. Neto MG, Silva LB, Grecco E, De Quadros LG, Teixeira A, Souza T, Scarparo J, Parada AA, Dib R, Moon R, Campos J. Brazilian Intragastric Balloon Consensus Statement (BIBC): practical guidelines based on experience of over 40000 cases.
2. Sallet JA, Marchesini JB, Paiva DS, Komoto K, Pizani CE, Ribeiro ML, Miguel P, Ferraz AM, Sallet PC. Brazilian multicenter study of the intragastric balloon. Obes Surg. 2004;14:991–8.
3. SAÚDE BMD. Vigitel Brasil 2014 Saúde Suplementar : vigilância de fatores de risco e proteção para doenças crônicas por inquérito telefônico. In: Saúde DdVdDeAnTePd, ed. Volume 1a edição -versão eletrônica. Brasília: Secretaria de Vigilância em Saúde. Agência Nacional de Saúde Suplementar, 2015:165.
4. Moura D, Oliveira J, De Moura EG, et al. Effectiveness of intragastric balloon for obesity: a systematic review and meta-analysis based on randomized control trials. Surg Obes Relat Dis. 2016;12:420–9.
5. Sander BQ, Galvao Neto M, Scarparo JIB, Schemberk JA Jr, Marchesini JCD, Grecco E, Barrichello S, Sander MQ. Intragastric balloon: conventional VS adjustable - First Brazilian comparative study. UEG Printer: Viena; 2016.
6. Sander BQ, Scarparo JIB, Galvao Neto M, Baretta G, Schemberk JA Jr, Fittipaldi-Fernandez RJ, Dib RA, Sander MQ. Intragastric balloon – a large Brazilian multicentric study of 4255 cases. Viena: UEG Week Printer; 2016.
7. Sander BQ, Galvao Neto M, Scarparo JIB, Fittipaldi-Fernandez RJ, Baretta G. Intragastric balloon: a Brazilian multicentric study of 3545 cases. 2015.
8. Sander BQ, Galvão-Neto M, Fittipaldi-Fernandez R, Baretta G, Scarparo J, Diestel C, et al. Op077: intragastric balloon in preparation for bariatric surgery patients. https://doi.org/10.1177/2050640614548983. https://www.ueg.sagepub.com/

Bariatric Surgeon Perspective on Bariatric Endoscopy and Intragastric Balloons: European Perspective

Rudolf A. Weiner, Sonja Chiappetta, and Sylvia Weiner

Introduction

In contrast to the USA, new technologies can be tested in Europe after a CE mark and ethical approval more easily in study series. This includes endoscopic bariatric and metabolic therapies in advanced stages of development and without regulatory approval by the U.S. Food and Drug Administration (FDA). Therefore, all new technologies were initially tested and introduced in the market in Europe or in Latin America in the past. However, for a long period, none of the endoscopic bariatric procedures were approved for use in the United States for bariatric indications. In discussing endoscopic procedures, it is helpful to separate them into metabolic and bariatric endoscopic interventions.

The longest and widest experience with intragastric balloons for weight loss is available in Europe. The field of bariatric endoscopy became relevant in Europe at the end of the last century (starting 1992), parallel to the introduction of minimally invasive surgery (MIS). The history and the situations were and are different from those in USA and other parts in the world.

Clinical and Diagnostic Aspects of the Disease

Role of Endoscopy in the Field of Bariatric and Metabolic Surgery

In Europe, many national regulations and specifications exist regarding the use of endoscopic techniques. In some countries, surgeons are not allowed to perform

R. A. Weiner (✉) · S. Chiappetta
Department of Obesity and Metabolic Surgery, Ospedale Evangelico Betania, Naples, Italy

S. Weiner
Department for Bariatric Surgery, Nordwest Hospital, Frankfurt am Main, Germany

© Springer Nature Switzerland AG 2020
M. Galvao Neto et al. (eds.), *Intragastric Balloon for Weight Management*,
https://doi.org/10.1007/978-3-030-27897-7_6

endoscopic approaches. Therefore, the indications for endoscopy before and after bariatric procedures are quite different. There are economic limitations in eastern Europe, which have an impact on the field of bariatric endoscopy as well.

In the Netherlands, for example, bariatric surgery is concentrated in hospitals with more than 500 cases per year in the past, and more than 1000 cases in the future. In this country, no endoscopic evaluation of the stomach is usually performed before bariatric procedures. Cost-effectiveness is the reason, caused by the fact that the surgeons are not allowed to perform upper endoscopy. The additional costs for a gastroenterologist are too high. This is at least one reason for such a strange situation. Under the same conditions, we can understand the arguments of a Dutch scientist that the endoscopic evaluation of the stomach before implantation of IGB is not necessary [1]. A comparable situation exists in Sweden.

In Germany, it is standard to investigate the upper GI tract, including testing for Helicobacter pylori infection, before any type of gastric surgery or endoscopic procedures. The entry to the endoscopic approach for surgeons is different. Some decades ago, all surgeons in Germany were allowed to perform upper and lower endoscopies, but in many hospitals, they lost this option and endoscopy became a domain of internal medicine specialists. But in the era of surgery for obesity and metabolic diseases, the importance of the endoscopic tools is increasing rapidly. In many private and public hospitals, a hard fight is necessary, to get back all the lost diagnostic and therapeutic options.

Especially in the management of complications, the endoscopic approach can save lives. In the era of sleeve gastrectomy, a leak in the His angle is a Damocles' sword over all procedures. Stent placement, sponge treatment, or other endoscopic maneuvers are necessary to manage this severe complication. Our wide experience was published early [2] and is documented in the book of Agrawal [3].

The Intragastric Balloon as a Weight Loss Procedure

In Europe, the intragastric balloon was introduced in 1992 as a weight loss procedure, being studied in clinical trials. The results of these are the basis for indications, techniques, and contraindications until now. We can separate the historical experiences in different time periods:

Era of Open Bariatric Surgery and First Balloon Trials: Before 1990
In the times of open bariatric surgery, endoscopy played no important role. The IGB was, for a long time, the only endoscopic bariatric procedure available.

Over the years, different balloon devices were tested, as they were thought to be promising and less invasive than surgery for the treatment of morbid obesity. By the end of the 1980s, several prospective, controlled studies reported that devices, such as the Ballobes and Garren–Edwards gastric bubbles, had no significant adjuvant effects for weight reduction. The reasons for this were the small volume of the balloon (220 ml for Garren—Edwards and 400 mL for Ballobes), the air-filling having no weight effect on the stomach walls, and the cylindrical shape. In addition, these devices had high rates of complications (26% gastric erosion, 14% gastric ulcer, 11% Mallory–Weiss tears) [4–9]. The use of the European balloons (Taylor, 1985; Ballobes bubble, 1988) ended in 1989. The manufacturer discontinued the production.

In this period, before the silicone IGB, other different types were used in small series. All these devices (some in a cubic form) were not stable, with several complications published, such as intestinal obstruction [6].

The Silicone Intragastric Balloon (SIB) was developed by Fred C. Gau in conjunction with INAMED Development Company (IDC) in 1986. In January 1996, the SIB was transferred from IDC to BioEnterics Corporation (BEC) and was renamed BioEnterics® Intragastric Balloon (BIB™) System. Later, this product was named the Orbera™ Intragastric Balloon System (Apollo Endosurgery Inc., Austin, TX, United States) and remains to be the mainly used product.

Others, like the ReShape Integrated Dual Balloon System (ReShape Medical, Inc., San Clemente, CA, United States) and the Obalon (Obalon Therapeutics, Inc.), still play a smaller role in Europe. The air-filled Heliogast balloon (France) was for a short period on the market.

First Trials and Congress Presentations: 1990–2000

Studies in the Netherlands

In early 1992, the FDA gave authorization for INAMED to export products to the Netherlands, and Mathus-Vliegen et al. started a clinical trial of the product. In 1995, an interim analysis of this trial's data was submitted to the FDA as part of the August 1996 Annual Report for the IDE and in 1997 the results of Mathus-Vliegen's 2-year study.

Forty-three patients participated in a 2-year trial involving 1 year of active balloon treatment and 1 year of balloon-free follow-up. After an initial 13 weeks of double-blind, sham-controlled balloon treatment, each patient had another three balloons at 13-week intervals. Energy-restricted diet, behavioral therapy, self-help groups, and exercise were part of the treatment program. Of the 43 patients in the study, 3 withdrew because of balloon intolerance, one patient did not cooperate at balloon placement, and another withdrew on his own request. Five patients had insufficient weight loss and were withdrawn from the study. Twelve patients experienced mild esophagitis related to medication and balloon intolerance and six patients experienced severe esophagitis. There were three gastric erosions. Balloon complications involved one gastric hemorrhage because of balloon removal, one balloon deflation in the stomach, and two balloons deflated and passed. Cultures of balloon contents were positive in 3 out of 15 balloons studied. All patients in the study lost an average of 26.3 kg; however, weight loss was only partially maintained in the balloon-free year with the average weight loss reduced to 14.7 kg. Initial balloon or sham treatment, active participation in a behavioral treatment or weight loss self-help group, the sex of the patient, or their initial starting weight had no influence on the amount of weight a patient lost. Mathus-Vliegen et al. concluded that in a multidisciplinary treatment, a 25 kg weight loss can be obtained by a moderately restricted diet combined with an intragastric balloon. Despite ongoing multidisciplinary treatment, this weight loss could only be partially maintained without other additional supportive measures [10, 11].

Studies in the UK

A small number of studies were done in the UK. In the study by P.J. Treacy in 1997 [12], patients had an average weight of 140 kg (103–223 kg) and an average body mass index (BMI) of 47.8 kg (41–66 kg). In all but one patient, insertion of the balloon was associated with a rapid initial weight loss of 2 kg per week (0.4–6.6 kg/week) over the first 4–8 weeks. The weight loss then slowed to an overall weight loss of 0.75 kg/week over the 26 weeks following insertion (0.2–2.6 kg/week). BMI was reduced to an average of 41.6 (36.9–49.5). The balloon was removed in one patient at week 25 due to severe reflux disease. At a 50-week assessment (25–58 weeks) using ultrasound and endoscopy, 9 balloons out of 11 had spontaneously deflated and passed. In the remaining two patients, the balloon had partially deflated at weeks 27 and 37. Of the nine collapsed balloons (seven patients), all but one patient had sensed balloon deflation by an increased ability to eat, reduced vomiting, and weight gain. The important message was that beyond a 6-month time span, the balloon is likely to spontaneously collapse, and its effects are lost.

Studies in Italy

Italy was the first European country to use more than thousands of balloons. Large series of national registries or multicenter studies were published after the year 2000.

Early in the 1990s, many Italian surgeons presented the first studies comparing balloon treatment with gastric banding, or as a single-stage procedure. Barratta et al. [13] showed the same initial weight loss after BIB and lap-band. The authors concluded that similar results can be obtained with the BIB System but only for a short period (up to 3 months).

Biondi et al. [14] compared the preliminary findings of laparoscopic restrictive surgery using an adjustable silicone band (laparoscopic adjustable esophagogastric banding – placing the band around the esophagus), with the use of the intragastric balloon. They concluded that the long-term weight loss was more satisfactory with the surgical procedure.

DeLuca et al. [15] concluded that a 25 kg weight loss could be obtained with a restricted diet combined with intragastric balloon. They found the endoscopic placement of the BIB System not to be difficult without general anesthesia. However, volume adjustment by intubation catheter was difficult because the valve position tends to be directly opposite to the side of the balloon visualized by the endoscope.

Doldi et al. [16] concluded after 37 cases that there are two problems related to the use of the BIB System: (a) the determination of the correct filling volume for each patient, and (b) poor patient compliance to dietary restriction.

Galloro et al. [17] reported the BIB System spontaneously deflated and passed with the stool in two cases. They concluded that the contraindications to the placement of the BIB System were the presence of *Helicobacter pylori* and peptic disease, which must be treated before undergoing BIB System placement. Absolute contraindications to the use of the BIB System were structural abnormalities in the esophagus or pharynx, large hiatal hernia, potential upper gastrointestinal bleeding conditions, congenital abnormalities of the gastrointestinal tract, and prior gastric or intestinal surgery.

Luppa et al. [18] compared the incidence of major and minor complications during the treatment of obese patients with the BIB System or LAP-BAND System. Fourteen patients were treated with the BIB System. The most common complications were vomiting and persistent nausea lasting 3–4 days (9/14 = 64%), abdominal cramps (3/14 = 21%), frequent belching (3/14 = 21%), and diarrhea (2/14 = 14%). Two patients had spontaneous deflation of the BIB System at 4 months with the balloon passing with the stool. No major complications were observed and there was no clinical evidence of esophagitis.

There were 26 patients treated with the LAP-BAND System. The average duration of surgery was 80 mins (range 45–180 mins). There were no conversions to open surgery. One patient had vomiting after surgery (1/26 = 38%). Constipation occurred in nine patients (9/26 = 35%). Pain was reported at the port site in seven patients (27%). Three (12%) patients experienced transitory dysphagia up to 1 month post-op. Two (2/26 = 8%) complained of asthenia and another two of hypoferremia.

Studies in Germany

Weiner et al. [19] published the results of the BIB System as a presurgical weight loss treatment for patients weighing more than 200 kg. Fourteen patients were treated. In 11 cases, the weight loss was successful with a range of 18–42 kg. Of the three unsuccessful patients, one could not tolerate the balloon, another had a spontaneous balloon deflation, and the third tended to eat sweets, which was cited as the cause for lack of weight loss. Weiner concluded that "the BIB System is a useful tool in reducing the preoperative body weight in extremely obese patients."

The largest series of super-, super-super-, and giant-obese patients were published by Weiner's group as well [20]. This is one of the largest reported cohorts of extremely obese patients, who underwent BIB insertion for the treatment of obesity. This treatment before a surgical procedure in such group of patients may reduce operative risks, regardless of whether the surgery is bariatric or not. It has been shown that a modest preoperative weight loss of 10–20% can reduce the complications of surgery. Preoperative weight loss is probably the most important method for reducing surgical risk in extremely obese patients. Conversion to open surgery was not necessary. The liver volume was markedly reduced.

The BMI loss or Excess Weight Loss (EWL) was related to the initial BMI or overweight (Fig. 6.1). Interestingly the percentage of patients who underwent bariatric surgery later was different in the BMI groups (Fig. 6.2). The complication rate was low (0.9% during insertion and 2.9% during removal). There was no mortality or severe complications noted.

Fig. 6.1 Mean BMI loss after intragastric balloon treatment (BIB): the trend line, the correlation coefficient, and the standard error of the mean (SEM) for each group are shown (Goethig et al. 2009)

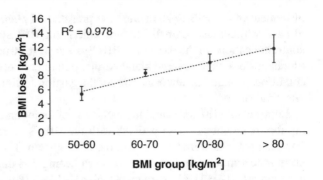

Fig. 6.2 Percentage of patients receiving subsequent surgery after intragastric balloon treatment (Goethig et al. 2009)

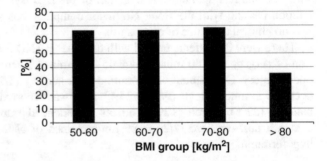

Period After the Year 2000

The use of IGB in medical weight loss centers is established in all European countries. It became a part of the European guidelines for interventional obesity treatment (Fig. 6.3). Based on the costs, which must be paid by the patient, the frequency of balloon treatments in western Europe is more common than in the eastern.

In contrast to most European countries, in Germany, the treatment in the hospital is covered by the insurance. The indications are the needed preoperative weight loss in super-obese patients, and the treatment in patients who are not candidates for weight loss surgery (e.g., AIDS).

In other countries, the balloon treatment is generally not covered by insurance companies. After the FDA-approval for Orbera in the USA, the number of balloon treatments has shown an increase in Europe as well.

Diabetes Type 2 and Metabolic Syndrome

After the fundamental studies of Francesco Rubino, duodenal exclusion became a therapeutic option for patients with type 2 diabetes mellitus.

The Endobarrier® (GI Dynamics, Lexington, Massachusetts, USA) is a duodenojejunal bypass sleeve comprising an impermeable sleeve of Teflon, anchored in the duodenal bulb by a nitinol crown with sharp barbs. This anchoring system is the Achilles' heel of the procedure. At first, the device was created as a weight loss procedure, then

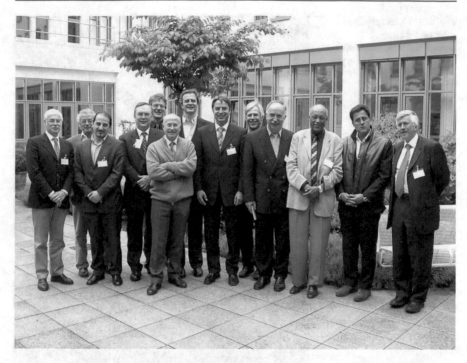

Fig. 6.3 European Consensus Conference of the EAES in 2004. From left to right: M. Garcia-Caballero (Spain), A. Fingerhut (France), F. Rubino (Italy), R. Tacchino (Italy), S. Sauerland (Germany), F. Favretti (Italy), M. Morino (Italy), R. Mittermaier (Austria), E. Neugebauer (Germany), R. Weiner (Germany), M. Belachev (Belgium), L. Angrisani (Italy), N. Finer (UK)

it showed remarkable metabolic effects, potentially manipulating the enteroinsulin system, becoming more of a metabolic procedure. Reports about liver abscess and perforation stopped the distribution of the device in Europe. If the anchoring system had been improved, it could have greater chances of becoming a real metabolic instrument. In our experience, the use of the device was stopped after a penetration into the gastroduodenal artery with massive hemorrhage (Figs. 6.4 and 6.5). The patient had to undergo laparotomy with a hemoglobin level less than 4 g% and survived.

Later, duodenal ablation or duodenal mucosal resurfacing was introduced as clinical trials in different European centers. In the Revita duodenal mucosal resurfacing procedure (Fractyl Laboratories, Cambridge, Massachusetts, USA), thermal ablation of the superficial duodenal mucosa is performed by using radio frequency. This was designed as a pure metabolic procedure. Final study results are not available at the moment.

The idea of Aspire® (Aspire Bariatrics; King of Prussia, USA) is completely different. It consists of a specially designed percutaneous gastrostomy tube, known as the A-Tube. The tube is made of silicone and is inserted in a fashion similar to that of a percutaneous endoscopic gastrostomy. Two weeks after insertion, the external portion of the tube is shortened, and a connector valve is attached. The connector

Fig. 6.4 Open revision after endobarrier complication: erosion of the gastroduodenal artery

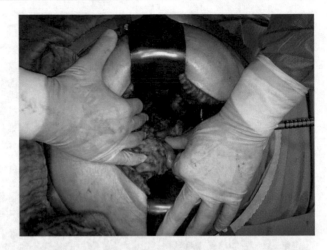

Fig. 6.5 Erosion of the spikes through the duodenal wall (same case in Fig. 6.4)

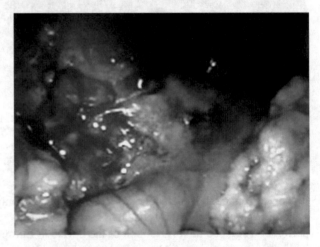

valve is flushed with the skin and is connected to the Aspire Assist device to allow aspiration of 30% of the ingested meal 20 mins after ingesting it. The first demonstration in Europe was in 2014 during the VIII Frankfurt meeting. There are small series published in some European countries. The largest experience exists in Czech Republic. No randomized controlled studies are available yet.

Indications and Contraindications of the Procedure

Intragastric Balloon

Indications

The use of IGBs in the treatment of morbid obesity appears to be effective when it is correctly applied. The balloon is not a modern panacea for obesity; the right selection of the patients and respect for the dietetic and behavioral rules are mandatory. In a multidisciplinary treatment, a 25 kg weight loss can be obtained with a moderately restricted diet combined with the IGB treatment. It is indicated to induce weight loss in patients whose obesity is not severe enough to make them candidates for surgery, to reduce the surgical risk, and to select patients for restrictive surgery when they lose weight with the balloon.

Contraindications

The detailed information about the first IGB studies between 1990 and 2000 is important. We learned from all mistakes. All major adverse events including death (s. FDA report 2017) happened, because the early lessons were not respected. Therefore, again the lessons, which we learned two decades before:

1. Use of the intragastric balloon is contraindicated in patients who had previous gastric surgery or diffuse peritonitis with fixation of the stomach.
2. Any inflammatory disease of the gastrointestinal tract including esophagitis, gastric ulceration, duodenal ulceration, cancer, or specific inflammation such as Crohn's disease.
3. Potential upper gastrointestinal bleeding.
4. Conditions such as esophageal or gastric varices, congenital or acquired intestinal telangiectasia, or other congenital anomalies of the gastrointestinal tract such as atresia or stenosis.
5. Large hiatal hernia.
6. Structural abnormality in the esophagus or pharynx such as a stricture or diverticulum.
7. Any other medical condition that could increase the risk of elective endoscopy.
8. Psychiatric disorders.
9. Alcoholism or drug addiction.
10. Patients unwilling to participate in an established medically supervised diet and behavior modification program.
11. Patients receiving aspirin, anti-inflammatory agents, anticoagulants, or other gastric irritants.
12. Patients who are pregnant or breastfeeding.

Aspire

Indications

Rare cases with the wish of uncontrolled eating, but psychological stable (no psychiatric diseases)

Contraindications

Same like IGB, in giant obesity with higher risks

Overstitch (Treatment of the Gastrojejunostomy)

Indications
In general dilatation of the gastrojejunostomy after "unbanded" Roux-en-Y gastric bypass; dumping syndrome; weight regain

Contraindications
Ulcerations in the gastrojejunal anastomosis

Endosleeve (Endoscopic Sleeve Gastroplasty)

Indications
Moderate weight loss needed or high-risk patients, after several previous abdominal surgeries

Endobarrier

Indications
Diabetes mellitus type 2 (ideal just before insulin therapy, Hba1c > 7, 5 g%); the preoperative weight loss for super-obese patients is not an ideal indication, because if complications occur, the management of perforations with bleedings and peritonitis in high BMI patients is extremely difficult.

Contraindications
Recurrent pancreatitis, obstructive jaundice, and all other contraindications for endoscopic implantation of devices

Duodenal Ablation

Indications
Experimental stage (diabetes mellitus type 2)

Endoscopic Maneuvers in the Management of Complications After Bariatric Surgery

In the era of Roux-en-Y gastric bypass, stenosis of the gastrojejunostomy was a common problem. The first choice is the balloon dilatation (Fig. 6.6), which is a solution in one to three sessions in most cases. Some patients need more sessions of dilatation, but surgical revision is rarely needed.

Currently, sleeve gastrectomy became the leading procedure worldwide. The main postoperative complications are bleeding, leak of the staple line, and stenosis.

Fig. 6.6 Endoscopic balloon dilation of the stenotic gastroenterostomy after gastric bypass

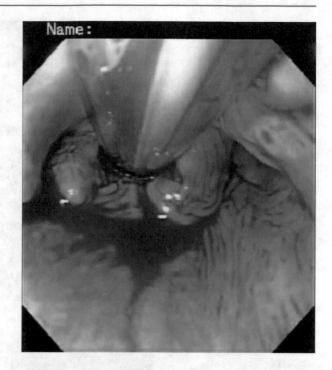

Fig. 6.7 OTS-Clip closing a chronic gastric fistula after RNYGB

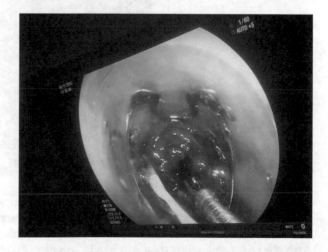

Intraluminal bleeding can be treated by classic endoscopic methods (injections, clips, etc.) [21].

Leak treatment is a domain of urgent endoscopy, using stents, clips (Fig. 6.7), sponges, or internal drainage (Fig. 6.8) including the placement of t-tubes. The indication and the management need highly specialized expertise, which is the criterion for a "bariatric endoscopist." If the leak is too large in diameter, then the over-the-scope (OTS) clip can pass through the hole and cannot be removed endoscopically (Fig. 6.9).

Fig. 6.8 Internal drainage of retrogastric abscess after sleeve gastrectomy

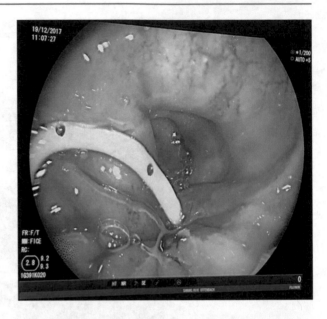

Fig. 6.9 Endoscopic closure of chronic fistula with OTS clip

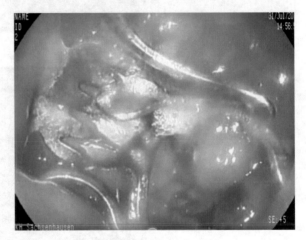

The sleeve stenosis (Fig. 6.10) can be treated by endoscopic dilatation as well. Two cases (one from Egypt and one from Germany) came as emergency cases into our department. They were unable to swallow any liquids after sleeve gastrectomy. Also, the upper endoscopy showed a nearly complete divided sleeve (Figs. 6.11 and 6.12). Using the endoscopic placement of a catheter to fill contrast medium under X-ray should demonstrate the option of dilatation. During this diagnostic maneuver, it became obvious that the sleeve was completely divided and that endoscopy would offer no solution. In these rare two cases, we had to perform laparoscopic revisional surgery immediately.

Our wide experience with chronic fistulas after sleeve gastrectomy (Fig. 6.13) taught us that if the early endoscopic treatment is done delayed or insufficient, the extreme open resection of the chronic fistula, sometimes multiple existing systems, may be necessary (Fig. 6.14).

Fig. 6.10 Mistake: three OTC clips placed in a too large leak – cause of a chronic fistula

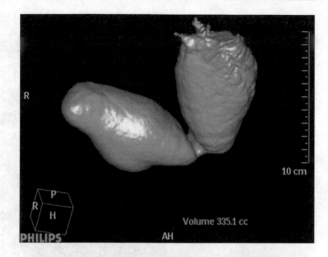

Fig. 6.11 Endoscopic view after sleeve gastrectomy: complete or uncomplete transection of the stomach during sleeve gastrectomy (Solution, see Fig. 6.12)

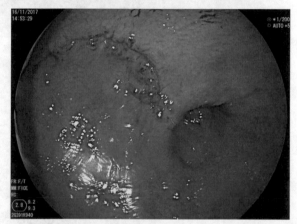

Fig. 6.12 Endoscopic maneuver with injection of contrast medium in potential sleeve stenosis, but it is complete divided sleeve

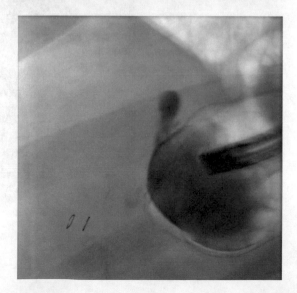

Fig. 6.13 Endoscopic
view on a small chronic
fistula after sleeve
gastrectomy

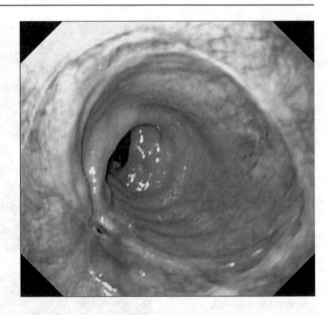

Fig. 6.14 Resected
fistulae with spleen after
complicated chronic sleeve
leak

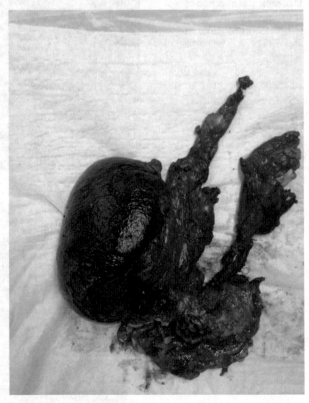

Discussion

The field of pharmaceutical-, surgical-, and endoscopic-induced weight loss is undergoing an explosion of new medications, techniques, and devices. A lot of these are geared toward endoscopic approaches rather than the conventional and more invasive laparoscopic or open approach. One such recent advance is the introduction of endoscopic suturing techniques. In contrast to North America, the balloon treatment is well established in Europe for more than 25 years.

Bariatric endoscopy became a specialized field during the last decade and more and more surgeons are interested in it. During the introduction of Overstitch procedure by Manoel Galvão Neto (Brazil) during the 8th Frankfurt Live-Surgery Meeting in 2014, Michel Gagner, a well-known international pioneer in minimally invasive surgery, was obviously very interested in the endoscopic maneuvers (Fig. 6.15).

Besides intragastric balloons, balloon dilatation of stenotic gastrointestinal anastomosis and sleeve, treatment of leaks by stents, clips, and sponge-treatments, the suturing techniques became a new role. The European experiences with endosleeve [22] and Overstitch [23] have just been published.

In contrast to the USA, Overstitch is used more frequently to treat patients with dumping syndrome after Roux-en-Y gastric bypass, rather than for weight regain. In our hospital, the first staple-line disruption was sutured using Apollo-OverStitch-technique, as discussed in C. Stier in 2016 (unpublished).

The situations in the European countries are quite different. The surgeons have, in many countries, no entry to the endoscopy. In some centers in the Netherlands and in Sweden, surgeons are not performing any endoscopic investigations before bariatric surgery. This is in contrast to our experiences [24] and European guidelines of the European Association for Endoscopic Surgery (EAES) [25]. The guidelines in 2004 expressed with a high degree of recommendation: "Upper gastrointestinal endoscopy or upper GI series is advisable for all bariatric procedures (GoR C), but

Fig. 6.15 Live transmission during eighth Frankfurt Meeting 2014. Michel Gagner watching Manoel Galvão Neto during the introduction of Overstitch in Germany

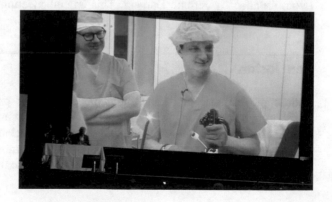

is strongly recommended for gastric bypass patients (GoR B)." The sleeve was, at this time, not a stand-alone procedure.

Therefore, we are wondering why with the balloon treatment, experienced gastroenterologists are performing the implantation of balloons under fluoroscopic guidance without a previous endoscopy, to assess the eligibility of patients and predicting adverse outcomes of balloon treatment [1].

In Germany, in some hospitals, the surgeons are allowed to perform upper endoscopies, but in some not. The first department for bariatric endoscopy only was developed by R. Weiner, C. Stier, S. Chiappetta, and O. Scheffel in 2014 (Sana Klinikum Offenbach a.M./Germany). Between 2001 and 2014, we used the interdisciplinary approach, which will hopefully be the future in Europe.

Besides the preoperative evaluation and intragastric balloon treatment, the main focus of postoperative management of complications changed in the last decades in Germany and in Europe:

1993–2000: Migration and erosion of the adjustable gastric banding. An endoscopic "band-cutter" was created by the Austrian company AMI. We used the endoscopic approach in cases of close to total migration successfully.

2000–2010: Stenosis of gastroenteroanastomosis after gastric bypass with balloon dilatation and diagnosing ulcerations

2010–present: Leaks and stenosis after sleeve gastrectomy. The increasing number of de novo Barrett's mucosa after sleeve gastrectomy led us to incorporate regular endoscopic controls of all sleeve patients in the future! This is an amazing perspective for the bariatric endoscopy.

The European Association for Endoscopic Surgery (EAES) is the platform of general and visceral surgeons for minimally invasive surgery, endoscopy, and ultrasound, comparable with Society of American Gastrointestinal and Endoscopic Surgeons (SAGES).

In contrast to the US, no "bariatric endoscopic" platform exists, like the Bariatric Endoscopy Task Force (BKAD) of the American Society of Gastroenterology. The European Chapter of International Federation for the Surgery of Obesity and Metabolic Disorders (IFSO) is endorsing every year the meeting "Non-invasiva" in Lyon, founded by Jerome Dargent. This annual meeting is focused on bariatric endoscopy only.

Conclusion

Endoscopic bariatric procedures hold the promise of providing the next major breakthrough not only in the management of overweight and obesity, but also in the treatment of diabetes mellitus type 2 and other weight-related diseases. A separation between weight loss procedures and metabolic procedures will be necessary in the future. These endoscopic procedures can offer a treatment in a safe, cost-effective, and minimally invasive fashion.

References

1. Mathus-Vliegen EMH. Is endoscopy really necessary for placing intragastric balloons? Obes Surg. 2018;28(1):169–75.
2. Scheffel O, Weiner RA. Therapy of stenosis after sleeve gastrectomy: stent and surgery as alternatives--case reports. Obes Facts. 2011;4(Suppl 1):47–9.
3. Weiner RA, El-Sayes IA, Weiner S. LSG: complications—diagnosis and management. In: Agrawal S, editor. Obesity, bariatric and metabolic surgery. Cham: Springer; 2016.
4. Edell SL, et al. Radiographic evaluation of the Garren gastric bubble. AJR Am J Roentgenol. 1985;145(1):49–50.
5. Diagnostic and therapeutic technology assessment. Garren gastric bubble. JAMA. 1986;256(23):3282–4.
6. Boyle TM, Agus SG, Bauer JJ. Small intestinal obstruction secondary to obturation by a Garren gastric bubble. Am J Gastroenterol. 1987;82(1):51–3.
7. Siardi C, et al. Treatment of obesity with gastric balloon. Minerva Dietol Gastroenterol. 1990;36(1):13–7.
8. Lindor KD, et al. Intragastric balloons in comparison with standard therapy for obesity--a randomized, double-blind trial. Mayo Clin Proc. 1987;62(11):992–6.
9. Bass DD, F L, Gottesfeld L. Antiobesity gastric balloon: an aid for achieving weight reduction. Experience with two types of balloons [Abstract], in 3rd Symposium on Obesity Surgery. 1987; Genova, Italy.
10. Mathus-Vliegen EM, Tytgat GN. Intragastric balloons for morbid obesity: results, patient tolerance and balloon life span. Br J Surg. 1990;77(1):76–9.
11. Mathus-Vliegen EM, Tytgat GN, Veldhuyzen-Offermans EA. Intragastric balloon in the treatment of super-morbid obesity. Double-blind, sham-controlled, crossover evaluation of 500-milliliter balloon. Gastroenterology. 1990;99(2):362–9.
12. Treacy PJ, M A W, Johnson AG. Use of the intragastric balloon for short term weight loss in patients with severe obesity. (Abstract) in Annual meeting of the Royal Australian College of Surgeons. 1997; Brisbane, Australia.
13. Barratta R, F L, Licciardello C, Finocchiaro C, Fullone F, Vigneri R, Luppa A. Adjustable silicone gastric banding and intragastric balloon: our experience. (Abstract) in 1st international symposium on Laparoscopic Obesity Surgery. 1999; Naples, Italy.
14. Biondi A, M A, Freschi M, Piazzini Albani A, Spinelli L, Vitellaro M, Novellino L, Laparoscopic adjustable esophagogastric banding Vs intragastric balloon. A preliminary experience. (Abstract) in 1st international symposium on Laparoscopic Obesity Surgery. 1999; Naples, Italy.
15. DeLuca M, L A, Formato A, De Palma G, Galloro G, Sivero L, Forestieri P. BioEnterics Intragastric Balloon (BIB) System: results of the follow-up and criteria of selection of the patients. (abstract) in 1st international symposium on Laparoscopic Obesity Surgery. 1999; Naples, Italy.
16. Doldi SB, D P F, Micheletto G, Bona D, Fichera G. Intragastric balloon in the treatment of obesity and morbid obesity: preliminary results. (Abstract) in 1st International Symposium on Laparoscopic Obesity Surgery. 1999; Naples. Italy.
17. Galloro G, et al. Preliminary endoscopic technical report of a new silicone intragastric balloon in the treatment of morbid obesity. Obes Surg. 1999;9(1):68–71.
18. Luppa A, S S, Villara S, Finocchiaro C, Baratta R, Licciardello C, Frittitta L. Short-Term Complications in Patients treated with BIB and/or LAP-BAND for Morbid Obesity. (Abstract) in 1st International Symposium on Laparoscopic Obesity Surgery. 1999; Naples, Italy.
19. Weiner R, Gutberlet H, Bockhorn H. Preparation of extremely obese patients for laparoscopic gastric banding by gastric-balloon therapy. Obes Surg. 1999;9(3):261–4.
20. Gottig S, et al. Analysis of safety and efficacy of intragastric balloon in extremely obese patients. Obes Surg. 2009;19(6):677–83.

21. Weiner S, et al. Anastomosis and suture insufficiency after interventions for bariatric and metabolic surgery. Chirurg. 2015;86(9):824–32.
22. Zorron R, et al. Endoscopic sleeve gastroplasty using Apollo Overstitch as a bridging procedure for superobese and high risk patients. Endoscopy. 2018;50(1):81–3.
23. Stier C, Chiappetta S. Endoluminal Revision (OverStitch (TM), Apollo Endosurgery) of the dilated gastroenterostomy in patients with late dumping syndrome after proximal Roux-en-Y gastric bypass. Obes Surg. 2016;26(8):1978–84.
24. Chiappetta S, et al. Incidental finding of GIST during obesity surgery. Obes Surg. 2015;25(3):579–83.
25. Sauerland S, et al. Obesity surgery: evidence-based guidelines of the European Association for Endoscopic Surgery (EAES). Surg Endosc. 2005;19(2):200–21.

Use of Intragastric Balloons in the Middle East: A Bariatric Surgeon Survey

7

Mousa Khoursheed, Jaber Al-Ali, and Abe Fingerhut

Introduction

The worldwide prevalence of obesity has nearly tripled between 1975 and 2016, when 39% of adults were overweight and 13% were obese [1]. Two populational studies have found that Kuwaiti adolescents showed the highest prevalence of obesity for both males (28.6%) and females (21.1%) when compared to eight other Arab countries [2].

Endoscopic bariatric procedures have emerged in the past few years; they have been adopted because they are reversible, repeatable, while less invasive and associated with lower costs compared with conventional bariatric surgery procedures. Such endoscopic bariatric procedures may have a place in weight-losing management, as well as filling the gap between medical and surgical procedures [3, 4].

The first intragastric balloon (IGB) device was introduced in the United States in 1985 (Garren–Edwards gastric bubble, GEGB) [5]. However, several side effects were observed, including gastric erosions (26%), gastric ulcers (14%), small bowel obstruction (2%), Mallory–Weiss tears (11%), and esophageal laceration (1%) [6].

Nonetheless, the simplicity of the IGB procedure would lead to its widespread role in obesity treatment and its applicability to various degrees of obesity. Notwithstanding, advances in device properties and procedural techniques are still needed to improve its safety and cost-effectiveness [7].

A systematic review including 26 primary studies ($n = 6101$) has shown that IGB devices are associated with a mean change in weight and BMI of 15.7 ± 5.3 kg and 5.9 ± 1.0 kg/m^2, respectively [8]. The most common complications observed were nausea/vomiting (23.3%) and abdominal pain (19.9%). Serious complications were

M. Khoursheed (✉) · J. Al-Ali
Kuwait Health Sciences Centre, Department of Surgery, Jabriya, Kuwait
e-mail: khoursheed@hsc.edu.kw; alalimd@hsc.edu.kw

A. Fingerhut
Medical University of Graz, Graz, Austria

© Springer Nature Switzerland AG 2020
M. Galvao Neto et al. (eds.), *Intragastric Balloon for Weight Management*,
https://doi.org/10.1007/978-3-030-27897-7_7

55

rare, including mortality (0.05%) and gastric perforation (0.1%). IGBs were associated with marked short-term weight loss with limited serious complications [8]. Weight loss is the result of increased satiety by the space-occupying device or delayed gastric emptying [9, 10]. Currently there are three IGB devices that have been approved by the U.S. Food and Drug Administration (FDA): The Reshape Integrated Dual Balloon System (Reshape Medical Inc., San Clemente, CA, USA), the ORBERA Intra-gastric Balloon System (Apollo Endosurgery Inc., Austin, TX, USA), and the Obalon intragastric balloon (Obalon Therapeutics, Carlsbad, CA, USA) [11].

To understand the current practice of IGBs in the Middle East Arab countries, we conducted a social media (Telegram) survey (Table 7.1) among all Arab country members of MENAC in December 2017. The results are described in this chapter.

Table 7.1 Space-occupying device survey

1. In which country you are working?
2. Years in practice
3. What is the estimated number of intragastric balloons (IGB) performed in your career?
4. How do you insert IGB (sedation/general anesthesia)?
5. Do you do IGB as OPD (Out-Patient Department) or as admission?
6. In water-filled IGB, do you add methylene blue?
7. Do you use the following IGBs? You can add more than one.
8. Do you do IGB for BMI < 27.5?
9. Do you do IGB prior to surgery in high risk patients if BMI > 50, 60, 70, never, other?
10. Do you do preoperative endoscopy?
11. If you find hiatus hernia would you insert IGB?
12. Do you do IGB for patients with peptic ulcer?
13. Do you do it for patients with IBD (Inflammatory bowel disease)?
14. Do you do IGB for patients with coagulopathy?
15. Do you do IGB for alcoholics or drug abuse patients?
16. What do you think the weight loss is on average after 3–6 months?
17. Do you think the 1-year IGB is better and the weight loss will be better?
18. Would you insert another IGB if the patient asks?
19. Do you think the IGB results are short-lasting?
20. If you think its short-lasting, do you tell your patient so?
21. Do you the IGB has metabolic effect?
22. How often patients complain of pain?
23. How often patients complain of nausea/vomiting?
24. Do you think GERD is major complication of IGB?
25. Do you prescribe PPI to all you patients till removal?
26. Did you have IGB migration?
27. How many times you had migrations and out of how many IGB inserted?
28. Which balloons you had migrations with and how many out of total?
29. Did you have IBG deflation? Specify type and number.
30. Did you have IBG small bowel obstruction? Specify type and number.
31. If so, specify which IGB and number out of total.
32. Did you need to operate to remove IGB due to intestinal obstruction?
33. If so, how often. Specify type of IGB.
34. Did you have gastric perforation after IGB?
35. If so, how many, specify which IGB.
36. What is the ideal filling volume of IGB?
37. What is the ideal content of IGB?
38. How do you remove IGB (sedation/general anesthesia)?
39. How often do you encounter early device removal?

Results

Of the 225 members who were contacted, 101 responded (44.8%), representing nine countries in the Middle East (Table 7.2); 48/101 (47.5%) of the participating surgeons had more than 15 years of practice.

Seventy-six of 101 (71.3%) replied that they were inserting IGBs at the time of the survey, while the remaining 25 were working in bariatric services that took care of patients with IGBs essentially to handle complications as part of multidisciplinary teams.

The total number of IGBs inserted by the participants was 16,503 (Table 7.3). The current practice of indications and contraindications, insertion and removal are shown in Table 7.4.

The rate of postoperative complications reported by participants is shown in Table 7.5. Device removal was necessary in <5%, 5–10%, and > 10% of cases, as reported by 32 (57.1%), 21 (37.5%), and three (5.4%) participants, respectively (Table 7.5). Balloon migration (0.3%), deflation (0.4%), small bowel obstruction (0.1%), reoperation for small bowel obstruction (0.08%), and gastric perforation (0.04%) according to the type of the balloon are shown in Tables 7.6, 7.7, 7.8, 7.9, and 7.10.

Table 7.2 Countries

	Number	%
Kingdom of Saudi Arabia	21	20.8
Egypt	8	7.9
Iraq	8	7.9
Jordan	6	5.9
Kuwait	27	26.7
Lebanon	4	3.7
Qatar	1	1
United Arab Emirates (UAE)	25	24.8
Yemen	1	1

Table 7.3 Types of balloons used by participants (60 responses)

	Number	%
Orbera	35	58.3
ReShape	4	6.7
Spatz	22	36.7
Ellipse	19	31.7
Obalon	14	23.3
Heliosphere	14	23.3
Silimed	1	1.7
Transpyloric shuttle	0	0
SatiSphere	1	1.7
Adjustable totally implantable intragastric prosthesis	1	1.7
Total IGB inserted	16,503	

Table 7.4 Preferred practice, indications, and contraindications

	Number	%
Sedation (IV/general)	44/25	63.7/36.3
OPD/admission	44/25	63.7/36.3
Methelyne blue (yes/no)	56/13	81.2/18.8
BMI < 27.5 kg/m^2 (yes/no)	16/51	23.9/76.1
For high BMI and high-risk patients prior to surgery (yes/no)	47/24	66.2/33.8
Preoperative endoscopy (yes/no)	46/21	68.7/31.3
Do in all patients with hiatus hernia (yes/no)	20/45	30.8/69.2
Do you do in patients with history of peptic ulcer (yes/no)	1/64	1.5/98.5
Do you prescribe PPIs until removal (yes/no)	53/13	80.3/19.7
Do you do IGB in patients with history of inflammatory bowel disease (yes/no)	20/44	31.2/68.8
Do you do IGB in patients with history of coagulopathy (yes/no)	9/54	14.3/85.7
Do you do for alcoholics and drug abuse (yes/no)	5/60	7.7/92.3
One-year IGB is better (yes/no)	23/43	34.9/65.1
Insert another IGB after removal	42/25	62.7/37.3
IGB is short- lasting (yes/no)	63/5	92.7/7.3
Information provided to patient that the effect is short	68/1	98.5/1.5
IGB has metabolic effect (yes/no)	20/48	29.4/70.6
Filling volume (<500, 500–700, >700)	6/50/2	10.3/86.2/3.4
Ideal content (liquid/air)	53/4	93/7
Removal (sedation/general anesthesia	35/24	59.3/40.7

Table 7.5 Complications

	Number	%
Pain (100%/50–100%/<50%)	13/32/19	20.3/50/29.7
Nausea vomiting (100%/50–100%/<50%)	26/28/10	40.6/43.8/15.6
GERD (yes/no)	23/41	35.9/64.1
Migration (yes/no)	21/44	32.3/67.7
Deflation (yes/no)	30/27	52.6/47.4
Small bowel obstruction (yes/no)	12/48	20/80
Reoperation for small bowel obstruction (yes/no)	11/44	20/80
Gastric perforation (yes/no)	8/52	13.3/86.7
Early device removal (<5%/5–10%/>10%)	32/21/3	57.1/37.5/5.4

Table 7.6 Balloon migration according to the manufacturer (total responses = 37)

	Number	%
Orbera	10	18.9
Ellipse	5	9.4
Heliosphere	1	1.9
Medsil	8	15.1
Obalon	1	1.9
Spatz	1	1.9
Uncertain	17	32.1
Total	53	100
Rate	53/16503	0.3

Table 7.7 Balloon deflation according the manufacturer (total responses = 44)

	Number	%
Orbera	20	28.6
Ellipse	8	11.4
Heliosphere	5	7.1
Medsil	3	4.3
Obalon	2	2.9
Spatz	2	2.9
Uncertain	30	42.9
Total	70	100
Rate	70/16503	0.4

Table 7.8 Balloon small bowel obstruction according to the manufacturer (total responses = 27)

	Number	%
Orbera	5	31.2
Ellipse	4	25
Heliosphere	0	0
Medsil	1	6.3
Obalon	0	0
Spatz	0	0
Uncertain	6	37.5
Total	16	100
Rate	16/16503	0.1

Table 7.9 Reoperation for small bowel obstruction according to the manufacturer (total responses = 25)

	Number	%
Orbera	5	38.5
Ellipse	3	23.1
Heliosphere	0	0
Medsil	0	0
Obalon	0	0
Spatz	0	0
Uncertain	5	38.5
Total	13	100
Rate	13/16503	0.08

Table 7.10 Gastric perforation according to the manufacturer (total responses = 23)

	Number	%
Orbera	5	71.4
Ellipse	0	0
Heliosphere	1	14.3
Medsil	0	0
Obalon	0	0
Spatz	0	0
Uncertain	1	14.3
Total	7	100
Rate	7/16503	0.04

Discussion

This survey, exploring the current practice of IGBs used in the Middle East Arab countries by members of MENAC from nine countries (82.2% from the Gulf region), showed that almost 80% used IGBs in their practice. Preoperative endoscopy was performed in all patients by 46 (68.7%) of participants. We found that IGBs were inserted for patients with hiatus hernia, history of peptic ulcer, inflammatory bowel disease, and history of coagulopathy, alcoholics and drug abuse in 30.8%, 1.5%, 31.2%, 14.3%, and 7.7% of patients, respectively. Our survey found that 43 of 66 responders (65.1%) did not believe that the 1-year balloon was better for weight loss, and 25 of 67 (37.3%) would not do sequential balloon insertions. Fifty-six (81.2%) participants mixed methylene blue with liquid-filled balloons and 53/57 (93%) preferred liquid-filled balloons. Overall complication rates were similar to other reports in the literature.

The IGB is one of the restrictive endoscopic procedures that induce gastric distension and satiety, delay gastric motility, and may have a hormonal effect. Due to its safety and simplicity, it has been adopted widely for patients who do not want or are unfit for surgery according to the established criteria for bariatric surgery. High-risk patients or those with severe obesity may also benefit from weight reduction prior to major bariatric surgery. Our survey found that 47/71 (66.2%) of inserted IGB were for high-risk patients or those with high BMI; 16/67 (23.9%) of participants insert IGB for patients with BMI < 27.5 kg/m^2, and 20/68 (29.4%) believe that the IGB has a metabolic effect.

The procedure can be done under sedation or general anesthesia [6]. Our survey showed that 44/69 (63.7%) and 35/59 (59.3%) preferred conscious sedation for insertion and removal, respectively. Forty-four out of 69 (63.7%) perform the procedure as an outpatient procedure.

As emphasized by several authors [12, 13] and the meta-analysis by Saber et al. [14], safety is an essential but debated issue. Relative and absolute contraindications for intragastric balloons include previous gastric surgery, hiatal hernia ≥ 5 cm, a coagulation disorder, a potential bleeding lesion of the upper gastrointestinal tract, pregnancy, alcoholism or drug addiction, severe liver disease, or any contraindication to endoscopy, and Crohn's disease [13].

Our survey found that preoperative endoscopy was performed in all patients by 68.7% of participants as well, IGBs were inserted for patients with hiatal hernia, history of peptic ulcer, inflammatory bowel disease, history of coagulopathy, alcoholics and drug abuse in 30.8%, 1.5%, 31.2%, 14.3%, and 7.7%, respectively.

Different types of balloon were used by participants, and some were using several different balloons in their practice. The Orbera balloon was inserted by 32 of 60 responders (58.3%). The long-term weight loss and the use of sequential balloon insertion has been addressed in previous reports [15, 16]. In our study, we found that 43 of 66 responders (65.1%) did not believe that the 1-year balloon was better for weight loss and 25 of 67 (37.3%) would not do sequential balloon insertions. Sixty-three of 69 (92.7%) believe that the weight loss is short-lasting and most (68/69, 98.5%) would inform their patients of this characteristic.

The major complaints of patients were epigastric pain and nausea/vomiting. In some patients, symptoms may last for more than a week [17] leading to voluntary removal of the balloon in up to 7% of cases [18]. We found that 53 (80.3%) of the participants prescribe proton pump inhibitors until removal. Device removal was necessary in <5%, 5–10% and > 10% of cases, as reported by 32 (57.1%), 21 (37.5%) and three (5.4%) participants, respectively.

Spontaneous deflation and balloon migration into the small bowel may occur [19]. Expert panel recommended that liquid-filled balloon should be mixed with methylene blue that can be absorbed and excreted with urine in the event of leakage [20]. In our survey, 56 of 69 (81.2%) participants said that they mixed methylene blue with liquid-filled balloons while (93%) preferred water-filled balloons. The filling volume used was 500–700 mL for 50 (86.2%) of the responders.

In our survey balloon migration, deflation, small bowel obstruction, reoperation for small bowel obstruction, and gastric perforation was found to occur in 0.3%, 0.4%, 0.1%, 0.08%, and 0.04% of patients, respectively.

Different Types of IGB on the Market and Their Use in the Middle East According to Our Survey

Orbera (BioEnterics)

This device is a spherical silicone elastomer device that is implanted endoscopically. Its capacity is up to 500–700 ml of saline, usually mixed with methylene blue. It is resistant to gastric acid up to 6 months.

Ten of the 53 patients who were reported to have migration had the Orbera balloon (18.9%). This relatively high prevalence might be attributed to the 58.3% rate of use by the participants in this survey. Furthermore, deflation, small bowel obstruction, reoperation for small bowel obstruction and gastric perforation was related to Orbera balloon in 28.6%, 31.2%, 38.5%, and 71.4% of total cases of complication reported, respectively.

Ellipse

The Ellipse™ (Allurion Technologies, Wellesley, MA, United States) does not require endoscopy or anesthesia for placement or removal. It can be simply swallowed under fluoroscopic visualization and once its position is confirmed in the stomach, the device is inflated with 550 mL of fluid. After 4 months, the balloon degrades, allowing the balloon to empty naturally and pass with stools [15].

Migration, deflation, small bowel obstruction, reoperation for small bowel obstruction, and gastric perforation were related to Ellipse in 9.4%, 11.4%, 25%, 23.1%, and 0% of cases reported, respectively.

Heliosphere Bag

The Heliosphere Bag (Helioscopie, Vienne, France) is positioned after diagnostic endoscopy. After placement, the balloon is slowly inflated with 840–960 cc of air; the final inflated volume is 650–700 cc, as the air is compressed [21].

Migration, deflation, small bowel obstruction, reoperation for small bowel obstruction, and gastric perforation rates were related to Heliosphere balloon in 1.9%, 7.1%, 0%, 0%, and 14.3% all cases reported, respectively.

Medsil

Medsil® intragastric balloon (Medsil, Russia) is positioned after diagnostic endoscopy. It is filled with up to 500–700 ml of saline usually mixed with methylene blue. The balloon should be removed after 6 months [16].

Migration, deflation, small bowel obstruction, reoperation for small bowel obstruction, and gastric perforation were related to Medsil balloon in 15.1%, 4.3%, 6.3%, 0%, and 0% of all cases reported, respectively.

Obalon

The Obalon intragastric balloon (Obalon Therapeutics, Carlsbad, CA) is a 250-mL gas-filled balloon that does not require endoscopy or anesthesia for placement. It is swallowed under fluoroscopic visualization and once its position is confirmed in the stomach, it is inflated with air. The balloon is removed endoscopically. A second balloon can be swallowed at 2 weeks and a third balloon at 4–8 weeks. Balloon should be removed endoscopically at 3 months [22, 23].

Migration, deflation, small bowel obstruction, reoperation for small bowel obstruction, and gastric perforation were related to Obalon insertion in 1.9%, 2.9%, 0%, 0%, and 0% of all cases reported, respectively.

Spatz

The Spatz Adjustable Balloon System (Spatz Medical, Great Neck, NY, United States) is a silicone liquid-filled balloon. It is attached to a filling catheter, which can be gripped endoscopically and allows volume adjustment of 400–800 ml. The balloon is removed after 12 months [24–26].

Migration, deflation, small bowel obstruction, reoperation for small bowel obstruction, and gastric perforation were related to Spatz balloon in 1.9%, 2.9%, 0%, 0%, and 0% of all reported cases, respectively.

ReShape Duo

The ReShape Duo® (ReShape Medical, San Clemente, CA, United States) is a liquid-filled double balloon device, inflated with 900 mL of saline, equally distributed to each of the two balloons. The liquid can be mixed with methylene blue. The balloon should be removed after 6 months. If one balloon ruptures or deflates, the other balloon usually remains inflated [27]. Only four members used this balloon in the Middle East, which accounts for 6.4% of the total of inserted IGB.

Transpyloric Shuttle

The Transpyloric Shuttle (BAROnova, Goleta, CA, USA) is made of a large spherical bulb attached to a smaller cylindrical bulb by a flexible tether. The cylinder is small enough to enter the duodenal bulb with peristalsis, and thus pulls the spherical bulb to the pylorus. The spherical bulb is too large to traverse the pylorus but occludes it intermittently to reduce gastric emptying. The device is delivered transorally via a catheter and removed endoscopically [28, 29]. This device has not been introduced to the Middle East and therefore was not reported in our survey.

SatiSphere

The SatiSphere (Endosphere, Columbus, OH, USA) is designed to delay transit time of nutrients through the duodenum. It consists of a 1-mm nitinol wire with pigtail ends and several mesh spheres mounted along its course, released in the duodenum and gastric antrum to conform to the duodenal C loop configuration and thereby become self-anchored. Device migration can occur, necessitating emergency surgery. The device delays glucose absorption and insulin secretion and alters GLP-1 levels [30]. Only one member used such a device in the Middle East.

Adjustable Totally Implantable Intragastric Prosthesis (ATIIP)

The (ATIIP)-EndogAst® (Districlass Medical, Saint-Etienne, France) is placed via a combined surgical and endoscopic procedure. The prosthesis is connected to a subcutaneous implantable system. It has a volume of 300 mL when inflated with air. It is placed with an endoscopic percutaneous gastrostomy technique followed by the deployment of a subcutaneous totally implantable system through a surgical procedure, thus designed to prevent migration and balloon adjustments [31]. Only one member used such a device in the Middle East.

Conclusions

With the efficiency and safety for the treatment of obesity by IGB showed by randomized clinical studies, these devices are widely used in the Middle East. Although compliance to the recommended indications and contraindications was not perfect, 63 (92.7%) of the participants believed that weight loss is short-lasting and almost two-thirds would not recommend sequential treatment. The majority used liquid-filled balloon mixed with methylene blue and the overall complications reported were similar to other reports in the literature.

Acknowledgments This study was made possible by the generous assistance and support of Arab country members of the Middle East and North Africa Chapter (MENAC) of the International Federation for the Surgery of Obesity and Metabolic Disorders (IFSO). We thank all of the participants.

Disclosures The authors have no conflict of interest.

References

1. World Health Organization: Obesity and Overweight, Fact Sheet No. October 2017. http://www.who.int/mediacentre/factsheets/fs311/en/.
2. Musaiger AO, Al-Mannai M, Al-Haifi AR, Nabag F, Elati J, Abahussain N, Tayyem R, Jalambo M, Benhamad M, Al-Mufty B. Prevalence of overweight and obesity among adolescents in eight Arab countries: comparison between two international standards (ARABEAT-2). Nutr Hosp. 2016;33(5):567. https://doi.org/10.20960/nh.567.
3. Bennett MC, Badillo R, Sullivan S. Endoscopic management. Gastroenterol Clin N Am. 2016;45(4):673–88. https://doi.org/10.1016/j.gtc.2016.07.005.
4. Sullivan S, Edmundowicz SA, Thompson CC. Endoscopic bariatric and metabolic therapies: new and emerging technologies. Gastroenterology. 2017;152(7):1791–801. https://doi.org/10.1053/j.gastro.2017.01.044. Epub 2017 Feb 10.
5. Benjamin SB, Maher KA, Cattau EL Jr, Collen MJ, Fleischer DE, Lewis JH, Ciarleglio CA, Earll JM, Schaffer S, Mirkin K, et al. Double-blind controlled trial of the Garren-Edwards gastric bubble: an adjunctive treatment for exogenous obesity. Gastroenterology. 1988;95(3):581–8.
6. Nieben OG, Harboe H. Intragastric balloon as an artificial bezoar for treatment of obesity. Lancet. 1982;1:198–9.
7. Kim SH, Chun HJ, Choi HS, Kim ES, Keum B, Jeen YT. Current status of intragastric balloon for obesity treatment. World J Gastroenterol. 2016;22(24):5495–504. https://doi.org/10.3748/wjg.v22.i24.5495.
8. Yorke E, Switzer NJ, Reso A, Shi X, de Gara C, Birch D, Gill R, Karmali S. Intragastric balloon for management of severe obesity: a systematic review. Obes Surg. 2016;26(9):2248–54. https://doi.org/10.1007/s11695-016-2307-9.
9. Sallet JA, Marchesini JB, Paiva DS, Komoto K, Pizani CE, Ribeiro ML, Miguel P, Ferraz AM, Sallet PC. Brazilian multicenter study of the intragastric balloon. Obes Surg. 2004;14(7):991–8.
10. Hodson RM, Zacharoulis D, Goutzamani E, Slee P, Wood S, Wedgwood KR. Management of obesity with the new intragastric balloon. Obes Surg. 2001;11(3):327–9.
11. Gleysteen JJ. A history of intragastric balloons. Surg Obes Relat Dis. 2016;12(2):430–5. https://doi.org/10.1016/j.soard.2015.10.074. Epub 2015 Oct 16.

12. Genco A, López-Nava G, Wahlen C, Maselli R, Cipriano M, Sanchez MM, Jacobs C, Lorenzo M. Multi-centre European experience with 315 intragastric balloon in overweight populations: 13 years of experience. Obes Surg. 2013;23(4):515–21. https://doi.org/10.1007/s11695-012-0829-3.
13. Yap Kannan R, Nutt MR. Are intra-gastric adjustable balloon system safe? Int J Surg Case Rep. 2013;4(10):936–8. https://doi.org/10.1016/j.ijscr.2013.07.025. Epub 2013 Aug 13.
14. De Castro ML, Morales MJ, Del Campo V, Pineda JR, Pena E, Sierra JM, Arbones MJ, Prada IR. Efficacy, safety, and tolerance of two types of intragastric balloons placed in obese subjects: a double-blind comparative study. Obes Surg. 2010;20(12):1642–6. https://doi.org/10.1007/s11695-010-0128-9.
15. Machytka E, Chuttani R, Bojkova M, Kupka T, Buzga M, Stecco K, Levy S, Gaur S. Elipse™, a procedureless gastric balloon for weight loss: a proof-of-concept pilot study. Obes Surg. 2016;26(3):512–6. https://doi.org/10.1007/s11695-015-1783-7.
16. Bužga M, Evžen M, Pavel K, Tomáš K, Vladislava Z, Pavel Z, Svagera Z. Effects of the intra-gastric balloon MedSil on weight loss, fat tissue, lipid metabolism, and hormones involved in energy balance. Obes Surg. 2014;24(6):909–15. https://doi.org/10.1007/s11695-014-1191-4.
17. Saber AA, Almadani MW, Zundel N, Alkuward MJ, Bashab MM, Rosenthal RJ. Efficacy of first-time intragastric balloon in weight loss: a systematic review and meta-analysis of random-ized controlled trials. Obes Surg. 2017;27:277–87.
18. Alfredo G, Roberta M, Massimiliano C, Michele L, Nicola B, Adriano R. Long-term mul-tiple intragastric balloon treatment--a new strategy to treat morbid obese patients refusing surgery: prospective 6-year follow-up study. Surg Obes Relat Dis. 2014;10(2):307–11. https://doi.org/10.1016/j.soard.2013.10.013. Epub 2013 Oct 25.
19. Dumonceau JM. Evidence-based review of the bioenterics intragastric balloon for weight loss. Obes Surg. 2008;18(12):1611–7. https://doi.org/10.1007/s11695-008-9593-9. Epub 2008 Jun 21. Review.
20. Schapiro M, Benjamin S, Blackburn G, Frank B, Heber D, Kozarek R, Randall S, Stern W. Obesity and the gastric balloon: a comprehensive workshop. Tarpon Springs, Florida, March 19–21, 1987. Gastrointest Endosc. 1987;33(4):323–7.
21. Forestieri P, De Palma GD, Formato A, Giuliano ME, Monda A, Pilone V, Romano A, Tramontano S. Heliosphere Bag in the treatment of severe obesity: preliminary experience. Obes Surg. 2006;16:635–7.
22. De Peppo F, Caccamo R, Adorisio O, Ceriati E, Marchetti P, Contursi A, Alterio A, Della Corte C, Manco M, Nobili V. The Obalon swallowable intragastric balloon in pediatric and adolescent morbid obesity. Endosc Int Open. 2017;5(1):E59–63. https://doi.org/10.1055/s-0042-120413.
23. Mion F, Ibrahim M, Marjoux S, Ponchon T, Dugardeyn S, Roman S, Deviere J. Swallowable obalon® gastric balloons as an aid for weight loss: a pilot feasibility study. Obes Surg. 2013;23(5):730–3. https://doi.org/10.1007/s11695-013-0927-x.
24. Russo T, Aprea G, Formisano C, Ruggiero S, Quarto G, Serra R, Massa G, Sivero L. BioEnterics Intragastric Balloon (BIB) versus Spatz Adjustable Balloon System (ABS): Our experience in the elderly. Int J Surg. 2017;38:138–40. https://doi.org/10.1016/j.ijsu.2016.06.013. Epub 2016 Jun 21.
25. Brooks J, Srivastava ED, Mathus-Vliegen EM. One-year adjustable intragastric balloons: results in 73 consecutive patients in the U. K. Obes Surg. 2014;24(5):813–9. https://doi.org/10.1007/s11695-014-1176-3.
26. Machytka E, Klvana P, Kornbluth A, Peikin S, Mathus-Vliegen LE, Gostout C, Lopez-Nava G, Shikora S, Brooks J. Adjustable intragastric balloons: a 12-month pilot trial in endo-scopic weight loss management. Obes Surg. 2011;21(10):1499–507. https://doi.org/10.1007/s11695-011-0424-z.
27. Ponce J, Woodman G, Swain J, Wilson E, English W, Ikramuddin S, Bour E, Edmundowicz S, Snyder B, Soto F, Sullivan S, Holcomb R, Lehmann J, REDUCE Pivotal Trial Investigators. The REDUCE pivotal trial: a prospective, randomized controlled pivotal trial of a dual intra-gastric balloon for the treatment of obesity. Surg Obes Relat Dis. 2015;11(4):874–81. https://doi.org/10.1016/j.soard.2014.12.006. Epub 2014 Dec 16.

28. Marinos G, Eliades C, Muthusamy V, Kobi I, Kline C, Narciso HL, Burnett D. First clinical experience with the transpyloric shuttle device, a non-surgical endoscopic treatment for obesity: results from a 3-month and 6-month study: SAGES; 2013. Abstract.
29. Unlu O, Okoh A, Yilmaz B, Roach EC, Olayan M, Shatnawei A. Endoluminal bariatric interventions: where do we stand? Where are we going? Acta Gastroenterol Belg. 2015;78(4):415–23. Review.
30. Sauer N, Rösch T, Pezold J, Reining F, Anders M, Groth S, Schachschal G, Mann O, Aberle J. A new endoscopically implantable device (SatiSphere) for treatment of obesity--efficacy, safety, and metabolic effects on glucose, insulin, and GLP-1 levels. Obes Surg. 2013;23(11):1727–33. https://doi.org/10.1007/s11695-013-1005-0.
31. Gaggiotti G, Tack J, Garrido AB, Palau M, Cappelluti G, Di Matteo F. Adjustable totally implantable intragastric prosthesis (ATIIP)-Endogast for treatment of morbid obesity: one-year follow-up of a multicenter prospective clinical survey. Obes Surg. 2007;17:949–56.

Part II
Devices

Liquid-Filled Balloon

8

Kais Assadullah Rona, Christopher DuCoin,
Marina S. Kurian, and Rachel Lynn Moore

Introduction

In 1985 the United States Food and Drug Administration (FDA) approved the Garren–Edwards Gastric Bubble (GEGB) as the first endoscopically implanted gastric balloon for the treatment of obesity [1]. In an era where procedures such as the Roux-en-Y gastric bypass and vertical banded gastroplasty predominated, the GEGB provided a novel, reversible, and less invasive alternative to complex bariatric surgery. Although the adoption of the first intragastric balloon was widespread across the world, the outcomes were less than optimal [2–4]. Weight loss was minimal, and the frequency of serious complications such as gastrointestinal obstruction and gastric ulceration was notable, leading to discontinuation of the device in 1988 [2–4]. Around the same time, different intragastric balloons were introduced (none of which were approved for use in the U.S.), such as the Taylor balloon (Mill-Rose Technologies, Cleveland, Ohio 1985) and the Ballobes bubble (DOT ApS Company, Denmark 1988). These devices varied in synthetic material (polyurethane *vs.* silicone), fill substance (air *vs.* saline), shape, size, and implantation duration. Despite

K. A. Rona
Department of Bariatric and Minimally Invasive Surgery, Tulane University,
New Orleans, LA, USA
e-mail: krona@tulane.edu

C. DuCoin
Department of Surgery, Tulane University, New Orleans, LA, USA
e-mail: cducoin@tulane.edu

M. S. Kurian
Department of Surgery, New York University, New York, NY, USA
e-mail: marina.kurian@nyulangone.org

R. L. Moore (✉)
Moore Metabolics & Tulane University, New Orleans, LA, USA
e-mail: rachel.moore@mooremetabolics.com

© Springer Nature Switzerland AG 2020
M. Galvao Neto et al. (eds.), *Intragastric Balloon for Weight Management*,
https://doi.org/10.1007/978-3-030-27897-7_8

these variations, weight loss outcomes remained suboptimal and similar complications to the GEGB were reported [5–8]. The disappointing clinical results of intragastric balloons set the stage for the convergence of international experts in a scientific meeting (the "Obesity and the Gastric Balloon: A Comprehensive Workshop") in 1987 aiming to identify a patient population that would benefit most from IGBs and to design the ideal balloon [9]. The conclusion of the conference set the standard for the ideal balloon, which would be spherical in shape, designed from silicone, filled with saline rather than air, up to a volume of 400–500 ml. Importantly, prior gastric surgery was to remain a contraindication to balloon insertion, and the device would be kept in place for 4–6 months.

The clinical application of IGBs was also established at the "1987 Obesity Congress", and these indications remain today. The balloons were to be used (1) in patients with a BMI between 30 kg/m² and 35 kg/m² as an adjunct to conservative weight loss measures, primarily in the form of diet and exercise; (2) in patients with a BMI greater than 40 kg/m² or a BMI greater than or equal to 35 kg/m², with at least one obesity-related comorbidity, who lack reasonable access to a bariatric center or are excluded based on increased intraoperative risk secondary to cardiovascular disease or other severe obesity-related comorbidities; and (3) in patients who are superobese (BMI >50 kg/m²) as a bridge to bariatric surgery to reduce surgical morbidity.

History and Outcomes of ORBERA

The Orbera® (Apollo Endosurgery, Inc., Austin, TX, USA) intragastric balloon (IGB), formerly BioEnterics Intragastric Balloon (Inamed, Santa Barbara, CA, USA), is an endoscopically placed spherical balloon that remains in the stomach for 6 months to induce weight loss, and is subsequently removed. It was first introduced in 1991 after the "1987 Obesity Congress" [1]. The conference aimed to develop the ideal gastric balloon while identifying a target population. Although not approved for use in Canada or the United States at the time, utilization of the BioEnterics Intragastric Balloon quickly spread across countries from South America to the Eastern hemisphere. Currently, there has been over 15 years of clinical experience with the Orbera® IGB, and it has been implemented in more than 80 countries worldwide with over 200,000 devices used [2].

In August 2015, the FDA approved the Orbera® device for use in the United States. The pivotal study was a multicenter, randomized, non-blinded trial that included 448 subjects to assess the safety and efficacy of the device. In addition, changes in weight and obesity-related comorbidities were compared in patients randomized to Orbera® IGB for 6 months with behavioral modification versus behavioral modification alone. Overall, mean % total body weight loss (% TBWL) was significantly higher in the Orbera® group at 6 months (10.1% vs. 3.3%), 9 months (9.1% vs. 3.4%), and 12 months (7.6% vs. 3.1%). There was no difference in the improvement of obesity-related comorbidities between the two groups. The rate of device and procedure-related serious adverse events was 10%, although there were no unanticipated adverse device effects or deaths.

Literature suggests that the combination of Orbera® IGB with lifestyle and dietary changes provides superior short-term weight loss relative to behavioral and dietary modification alone [3]. The Italian experience reported a mean percent excess weight loss of 33.9 after 6 months in 2515 patients that had undergone treatment with Orbera® IGB [4]. In a recent randomized trial by Courcoulas et al., improved weight loss outcomes were demonstrated in patients who underwent Orbera® and lifestyle change in comparison to those who underwent lifestyle change alone [2]. Their study showed significantly higher weight loss at 6 months (10% TBWL *vs.* 3.3% TBWL, $P < 0.001$) in the Orbera® treatment arm. Improved weight loss was maintained at 3 and 6 months post balloon removal. Similar results have been reported in other prospective studies [5–7]. Despite this, long-term data on weight loss maintenance is unknown [8, 9].

The Device

The Orbera® balloon is made of an inert, non-toxic, and soft silicone viscoelastic polymer. The outer surface of the balloon is resistant to friction against the gastric mucosa, limiting focal point irritation. Unlike previous balloons, which were filled with air, the Orbera® balloon is filled with saline allowing it to float freely within the gastric lumen and preferentially remain in the body of the stomach. The expansible design can hold a wide volume of saline ranging from 400 cc (diameter of 9.14 cm) up to 700 cc (diameter of 11 cm). The volume of the balloon cannot be adjusted once it has been filled. Additionally, it is radiopaque and easily identified on radiography.

Although the mechanism of action of the Orbera® IGB has not been fully elucidated, it appears to be multifactorial and related to both physiological and neurohormonal factors. First, the inflated balloon acts as an artificial bezoar preloading the stomach and decreasing the size of the gastric reservoir to induce early satiety [10]. A second mechanism involves alterations in gut hormones and gastric motility. In a study by Mion et al., plasma ghrelin levels decreased and gastric emptying time was delayed in patients following IGB placement [11]. Other studies have demonstrated a similar effect on gastric motility [12, 13]. Despite this, the data is inconsistent, and it remains unclear whether these potential changes in gut hormone levels and gastric emptying actually correlate with weight reduction.

Indications

Indications for the use of Orbera® IGB differ in the US and internationally. In the United States, implantation is indicated as an adjunct to weight reduction for patients with a BMI of ≥ 30 Kg/m^2 or ≤ 40 Kg/m^2 in conjunction with an intensive supervised diet and lifestyle modification program. The presence of obesity-related comorbidities is not required. A failed attempt at conservative weight loss measures including supervised diet, behavior modification regimens, and exercise programs should precede placement of the Orbera® IGB. Body mass index requirements are less stringent internationally. In Europe, Canada, Brazil, and Australia, Orbera® use is expanded to overweight patients with a BMI > 27 Kg/m².

Contraindications

Knowledge of absolute and relative contraindications of Orbera® IGB implantation is important in optimizing patient safety and minimizing risk. Common absolute contraindications include:

- Presence of more than one intragastric balloon simultaneously
- Prior gastrointestinal or bariatric surgery
- Presence of a large hiatal hernia (>5 cm) or a smaller hiatal hernia with intractable gastroesophageal reflux (GERD) symptoms
- Severe esophagitis (Los Angeles Grade C and D)
- Structural esophageal or pharyngeal abnormalities such as esophageal stricture or diverticulum
- Esophageal motility disorders (i.e., achalasia)
- Severe coagulopathy, hepatic insufficiency, or cirrhosis
- Presence of a gastric mass
- Inflammatory conditions of the gastrointestinal tract (i.e., esophagitis, gastric ulceration, duodenal ulceration)
- Conditions predisposing to potential upper gastrointestinal bleeding (including esophageal/gastric varices, congenital or acquired intestinal telangiectasias)
- Pregnancy or desire to become pregnant
- Patients with known or suspected allergies to materials contained in Orbera®
- Any contraindication to endoscopy
- Psychiatric illness or disorder, which prevents the patient from complying to follow-up visits and removal of the device after 6 months

Relative contraindications include Crohn's disease, previous abdominal surgery, presence of a hiatal hernia, use of nonsteroidal and anti-inflammatory medication, uncontrolled psychiatric disease, or inability/unwillingness to comply with prescribed anti-secretory medications.

Procedure and Patient Management

All patients who are being considered for Orbera® IGB placement should undergo a thorough evaluation of medical history and a full physical examination. Assessment for any swallowing dysfunction/disorders or esophageal disorder should be performed. Pre-procedure workup includes appropriate blood tests (basic metabolic panel, liver function panel, lipid studies, coagulation function) and an electrocardiogram. Patients with gastroesophageal reflux require anti-secretory medications prior to Orbera® implantation. With respect to preoperative counseling, it is important to establish realistic patient expectations and stress the critical role of lifestyle change and dietary modification in conjunction with the IGB for successful outcomes.

The Orbera® balloon is supplied attached to the Placement Catheter Assembly (PCA), a silicone catheter that is connected on one end to a sheath containing the collapsed balloon and on the other end to a Luer-Lock connector that attaches the filling system. The filling system includes a fill tube, filling valve, and an IV spike. If the device has any evidence of damage, it should not be used, and a new device should be obtained.

The procedure begins with upper gastrointestinal endoscopy to evaluate gastro-esophageal anatomy and possible contraindications to intragastric balloon placement. The endoscope is then removed upon completion. The Placement Catheter Assembly (PCA) with the internal guidewire is carefully inserted into the esophagus and ideally positioned in the stomach. The endoscope is then reinserted alongside the catheter and the PCA is guided beyond the lower esophageal sphincter and into the stomach. Once the catheter is positioned, the guidewire is removed. The following step is filling of the balloon with sterile saline. It is important to maintain the position of the catheter alongside the endoscope, so it is not pulled back during inflation of the balloon. The filling system spike is inserted into a sterile saline bag. A 50 cc syringe and the fill tube (using the Luer-Lock connector) is then attached to the filling system valve. The Orbera® balloon can be filled with 400 cc to a maximum of 700 cc of saline. It should not be filled with any less volume than 400 cc or more volume than 700 cc, as this can lead to serious and life-threatening complications.

In a meta-analysis of 44 studies (5549 patients) by Kumar et al., there was no significant correlation between balloon-filling volumes and % total body weight loss at 6 months although larger filling volumes were less likely to migrate [14]. All the included studies used filling volumes of 500–700 cc. The current recommendation is filling volumes of 500 to 650 cc. Once the balloon is filled with the desired volume of saline, the fill kit is removed from the fill tube. The balloon valve is sealed by drawing back on the fill tube with the syringe to produce suction on the placement catheter. Finally, the balloon is separated from the fill tube by gently pulling the tube against the lower esophageal sphincter or tip of the endoscope.

Knowledge of the anticipated physiological responses to the Orbera® device allows the clinician to optimize patient tolerability while minimizing adverse symptoms. Common post-procedure side effects include nausea, vomiting, and abdominal pain. The majority of patients (59.7%) have mild symptoms, while 5.8% may experience severe symptoms. To aid in management of typical postoperative symptoms a treatment protocol including anti-emetics, proton-pump inhibitors, and close patient monitoring is recommended. Proton-pump inhibitors should be started 2 weeks prior to IGB placement and continued through the removal of the device. Aggressive management of nausea with anti-emetics and anticholinergics should be planned on the day of the procedure and continued for 2–5 days, then used on an as needed basis for 1 week following placement of the balloon. Adequate hydration is of utmost importance during and after the procedure. Goal fluid intake is 1.5 liters over a 24-hour period. The clinician is expected to contact the patient at 24 hours and daily for 1 week to assess both fluid intake and symptoms. If a patient is experiencing severe symptoms and unable to maintain adequate fluids, prompt evaluation of the patient and intervention is crucial.

Although IGB placement is a relatively low risk procedure, rare serious complications including visceral perforation, major gastric hemorrhage, bowel obstruction, pancreatitis, and resulting mortalities have been reported [15–17]. Five deaths related to the Orbera balloon were reported to the FDA in 2016 although the true incidence rate of patient death is unknown. In a systematic review of mostly fluid-filled IGBs, the rate of gastric perforation and mortality was 0.1% and 0.05%, respectively [18]. Recently, in February 2017, an updated FDA-issued alert was published describing the phenomena of spontaneous balloon over-inflation and pancreatitis shortly following IGB placement. Thus, knowledge of proper insertion, filling, and removal techniques in addition to its possible complications is critical.

In the U.S., The Orbera® device is designed to remain in place for a maximum of 6 months. Use of Orbera® beyond 6 months increases the risk of balloon deflation with subsequent morbidity, including gastrointestinal obstruction and mortality. Earlier removal is recommended in patients who become pregnant after balloon placement, are undergoing planned surgery, or develop intolerance to the device and those with a deflated balloon. Removal of the balloon is done under sedation with endoscopy according to general hospital protocol. The filled balloon is visualized endoscopically, and a needle instrument is guided down the working channel of the endoscope. The balloon is then punctured, and suction tubing is pushed through the balloon shell. Once the needle is removed, suction is applied and the fluid from the balloon is evacuated. The suction tubing is subsequently removed from the working channel, and a two-pronged grasper is inserted and used to grasp the balloon. With a firm grip on the balloon, it is slowly extracted up to the esophagus and removed.

Aftercare Platform

Following payment for the procedure, which at this time is not covered by insurance, patients are provided personalized aftercare education for up to 6 months after device removal. A unique aftercare platform that functions to provide post-procedure support to patients is the Orbera® COACH. This is a mobile application that provides patients with live personal and group sessions with dietitian coaches, motivational strategies, educational content, and a means to record and track dietary information. For example, the Orbera® COACH allows online and app-based weight tracking and picture-based meal tracking to give patients up-to-date and comprehensive data regarding their progression. Furthermore, among other things, the platform contains detailed nutritional content, meal recipes, and lifestyle tips. Primary providers are also able to access the platform and monitor a patient's weight loss trends. Other options include having the practice dietitian follow the patient with a year of aftercare.

References

1. Gleysteen JJ. A history of intragastric balloons. Surg Obes Relat Dis. 2016;12:430–5.
2. Courcoulas A, Abu Dayyeh BK, Eaton L, Robinson J, Woodman G, Fusco M, et al. Intragastric balloon as an adjunct to lifestyle intervention: a randomized controlled trial. Int J Obes. 2017:1–7. https://doi.org/10.1038/ijo.2016.229.
3. Imaz I, Martinez-Cervell C, Garcia-Alvarez EE, Sendra-Gutierrez JM, Gonzalez-Enriquez J. Safety and effectiveness of the intragastric balloon for obesity. A meta-analysis. Obes Surg. 2008;18(7):841–6.
4. Genco A, Bruni T, Doldi SB, Forestieri P, Marino M, Busetto L, et al. BioEnterics intragastric balloon: the Italian experience with 2,515 patients. Obes Surg. 2005;15:1161–4.
5. Fuller NR, Pearson S, Lau NS, Wlodarczyk J, Halstead MB, Tee H, et al. An intragastric balloon in the treatment of obese individuals with metabolic syndrome: a randomized controlled study. Obesity. 2013;21(8):1561–70.
6. Herve J, Wahlen CH, Schaeken A, Dallemagne B, Dewandre JM, Markiewicz S, et al. What becomes of patients one year after the intragastric balloon has been removed? Obes Surg. 2005;15(6):864–70.
7. Mathus-Vliegen EM, Tytgat GN. Intragastric balloon for treatment-resistant obesity: safety, tolerance, and efficacy of 1-year balloon treatment followed by a 1-year balloon-free follow-up. Gastrointest Endosc. 2005;61(1):19–27.
8. Dastis NS, Francois E, Deviere J, Hittelet A, Ilah Mehdi A, Barea M, et al. Intragastric balloon for weight loss: results in 100 individuals followed for at least 2.5 years. Endoscopy. 2009;41(7):575–80.
9. Kotzampassi K, Grosomanidis V, Papakostas P, Penna S, Eleftheriadis E. 500 intragastric balloons: what happens 5 years thereafter? Obes Surg. 2012;22(6):896–903.
10. Nieben OG, Harboe H. Intragastric balloon as an artificial bezoar for treatment of obesity. Lancet. 1982;1(8265):198–9.
11. Mion F, Napoleon B, Roman S, Malvoisin E, Trepo F, Pujol B. Effects of intragastric balloon on gastric emptying and plasma ghrelin levels in non-morbid obese patients. Obes Surg. 2005;15(4):510–6.
12. Su HJ, Kao CH, Chen WC, Chang TT, Lin CY. Effect of intragastric balloon on gastric emptying time in humans for weight control. Clin Nucl Med. 2013;38(11):863–8.
13. Gomez V, Woodman G, Abu Dayyeh BK. Delayed gastric emptying as a proposed mechanism of action during intragastric balloon therapy: results of a prospective study. Obesity. 2016;24(9):1849–53.
14. Kumar N, Bazerbachi F, Rustagi T, McCarty TR, Thompson CC, Galvao Neto MP, et al. The influence of the orbera intragastric balloon filling volumes of weight loss, tolerability, and adverse events: a systematic review and meta-analysis. Obes Surg. 2017;27(9):2272–8.
15. Granek RJ, Hii MW, Ward SM. Major gastric haemorrhage after intragastric balloon insertion: case report. Obes Surg. 2018;28:281–4.
16. Yorke E, Switzer NJ, Reso A, et al. Intragastric balloon for management of severe obesity: a systematic review. Obes Surg. 2016;26:2248–54.
17. Tate CM, Geliebter A. Intragastric balloon treatment for obesity: review of recent studies. Adv Ther. 2017;34(8):1859–187.
18. Yorke E, Switzer NJ, Reso A, Shi X, de Gara C, Birch D, et al. Intragastric balloon for management of severe obesity: a systematic review. Obes Surg. 2016;26(9):2248–54.

Adjustable Liquid-Filled Balloon: An Overview

9

Eduardo N. Usuy Jr., Ricardo José Fittipaldi-Fernandez, and Vitor Ottoboni Brunaldi

Introduction

Treating obesity and overweight using intragastric balloons has been well established for a long time since their safety and efficacy have been undoubtedly shown [1]. The volume of the traditional nonadjustable balloon is determined at the moment of the implantation and varies from 400 to 700 ml [2]. However, once it has been filled, it cannot be adjusted, therefore the dimension of the balloon will remain the same until the end of the treatment. The maximum indwelling time for the traditional device is 180 days. Then, it must be removed.

About 2 years ago, Brazil approved the use of the liquid-filled adjustable intragastric balloon (Spatz®). The currently available device is the third generation, which is much safer and easier to handle than the earlier versions. Certain features were set as targets for the third-generation intragastric balloon to possess:

1. Capable of holding a variable volume of filling liquid (400–700 ml)
2. Liquid-filled
3. Presence of a radiopaque mark (for follow-up control)
4. Made of durable-resistant material (to prevent leakage)

E. N. Usuy Jr.
Department of Gastroenterology and Bariatric Surgery, Gástrica Clinic, Florianópolis, SC, Brazil
e-mail: usuy@usuy.com.br

R. J. Fittipaldi-Fernandez (✉)
Department of Bariatric Endoscopy, Endogastro Rio Clinic, Rio de Janeiro, RJ, Brazil

V. O. Brunaldi
Endoscopy Unit of the Department of Gastroenterology, (Hospital das Clínicas da Faculdade de Medicina da Universidade de São Paulo), University of São Paulo (Universidade de São Paulo), São Paulo, SP, Brazil
e-mail: vitor.brunaldi@usp.br

© Springer Nature Switzerland AG 2020
M. Galvao Neto et al. (eds.), *Intragastric Balloon for Weight Management*,
https://doi.org/10.1007/978-3-030-27897-7_9

5. Smooth-surfaced (to hinder ulceration)

In regard to the first item, the Spatz® balloon is superior to the standard balloon because the endoscopist can control its volume throughout the period of treatment, not only at the moment of implantation [3]. However, concerning the last item, the traditional device seems better than the Spatz® since the latter has a permanent "tail"-shaped catheter used to adjust the volume of the balloon [4].

Differences of the Spatz® Adjustable Balloon

Post-Implantation Control The volume of the Spatz® balloon can be increased or diminished at any time of the treatment.

- The volume of the balloon can be reduced if a patient is suffering from severe adaptation symptoms (uncontrolled vomiting or vomiting for more than 7 days). The endoscopist may deflate 100–300 ml to alleviate symptoms, thus allowing the continuity of the treatment precluding early removal. Studies from the literature and our personal experience demonstrate that all patients who agree with the partial deflation continue the treatment until the end, thereby significantly reducing early balloon removal rate, which is around 5% for the standard balloon [5–7].
- The Spatz® balloon may be filled up either at a scheduled date or when the patient no longer reports improved satiety. The increase in balloon volume enhances the restriction of food intake and the feeling of satiety. Some studies have shown that patients who adjust the balloon in the sixth month lose more weight from the sixth to the twelfth month compared to patients who do not [3, 5–7]. Therefore, that is our daily practice for the treatment with Spatz®.

Maximum Indwelling Time of 1-Year Apparently, the duration of treatment of 12 months does not lead to a greater overall weight loss compared to the 6-month therapy [4]. However, the weight loss is sustained for 1 year whereas patients who undergo the 6-month treatment usually regain some of the lost weight at the twelfth month after implantation (6 months after balloon removal). Furthermore, the longer period grants more time for the patient to adapt to the lifestyle modifications which are central to achieve success.

Results

The loss of weight associated with the adjustable balloon after 1 year is similar to that after 6 months with the conventional balloon [1–4]. Table 9.1 outlines the results from the available studies assessing weight loss with the Spatz®.

Of note, some studies suggest a trend toward greater weight loss in the group who undergo an increase in the volume of the balloon in the middle of the treatment,

Table 9.1 Results from studies assessing the effectiveness of the adjustable liquid-filled balloon

Study	Total weight loss (%)	Excess weight loss (%)	Total weight loss (kg)
Machytka et al. (2011) [3]	–	48.8	24.4
Genco et al. (2013) [4]	–	56.7	–
Machytka et al. (2014) [5]	15.9	40.1	17.2
Brooks et al. (2014) [6]	20.1	45.8	24.0
Machytka et al. (2015) [7]	15.2^a/18.2^b	39.7^a/43.4^b	16.4^a/20.4^b
Fittipaldi-Fernandez et al. (2016)^c	17.97^a/18.14^b	55.54^a/60.62^b	19.39^a/19.46^b

^{a}No balloon volume increase during treatment
^{b}Balloon volume increase during treatment
^{c}Data yet to publish

compared to the group with no adjustment. That trend, however, did not reach statistical difference ($p > 0.05$) [5–7].

Complications

The adverse events related to the Spatz3® balloon are the same as those from the traditional model [1]. However, we noticed a higher incidence of gastric ulcers, usually caused by the overpressure of the "tail"-shaped catheter and located at the *incisura angularis* [4]. In the author's casuistic, the incidence is 2.46% for such ulcers. However, the ulcerations are usually shallow, asymptomatic, and easy to manage. There was no statistical difference in regard to other complications comparing the traditional and the adjustable balloons. Finally, there were no cases of perforations, hemorrhages, or other serious adverse events in our series.

Conclusion

The adjustable intragastric balloon is a promising device to treat overweight and obesity. It carries similar weight loss to the traditional balloon but is able to sustain it for 12 months. It may also reduce the incidence of early removal rates which has an acceptable safety profile.

References

1. Sallet JA, Marchesini JB, Paiva DS, Komoto K, Pizani CE, Ribeiro ML, et al. Brazilian multi-center study of the intragastric balloon. Obes Surg. 2004;14(7):991–8.
2. Genco A, Bruni T, Doldi SB, Forestieri P, Marino M, Busetto L, et al. BioEnterics intragastric balloon: the Italian experience with 2,515 patients. Obes Surg. 2005;15(8):1161–4.
3. Machytka E, Klvana P, Kornbluth A, Peikin S, Mathus-Vliegen LE, Gostout C, et al. Adjustable intragastric balloons: a 12-month pilot trial in endoscopic weight loss management. Obes Surg. 2011;21(10):1499–507.

4. Genco A, Dellepiane D, Baglio G, Cappelletti F, Frangella F, Maselli R, et al. Adjustable intra-gastric balloon vs non-adjustable intragastric balloon: case-control study on complications, tolerance, and efficacy. Obes Surg. 2013;23(7):953–8.
5. Machytka E, Brooks J, Buzga M, Mason J. One year adjustable intragastric balloon: safety and efficacy of the Spatz3 adjustable balloons. F1000 Research. 2014;3:203.
6. Brooks J, Srivastava ED, Mathus-Vliegen EM. One-year adjustable intragastric balloons: results in 73 consecutive patients in the U.K. Obes Surg. 2014;24(5):813–9.
7. Machytka E, Marinos G, Kerdahi RF, Srivastava ED, AlLehibi A, Mason J, Buzga M, Brooks J. Spatz adjustable balloons: results of adjustment for intolerance and for weight loss plateau. Gastroenterology. 2015;148(Issue 4, Supplement 1):S-900.

Liquid-Filled Double Balloon: U.S. Experience

10

Jaime Ponce

Introduction

The saline-filled double intragastric balloon (Reshape Medical, San Clemente, California, United States) is a weight loss system that consists of two independently inflated, noncommunicating, silicone balloons tethered to a central silicone shaft. Each balloon can be inflated independently with 375–450 mL of saline solution (manufacturer recommends that patients of height shorter than 64 inches inflate with 375 mL and taller patients use 450 mL on each balloon) and remains in the stomach for 6 months (Fig. 10.1).

Placement and Removal Techniques

Placement involves doing an initial upper endoscopy screening. Then a guide wire is placed through the working channel of the scope, leaving the distal tip of the wire in the proximal duodenum. The scope is withdrawn, leaving the guide wire in place. Then the balloons with the delivery catheter are inserted through the guide wire all the way to the 50 cm mark. It is important to always use plenty of lubrication, adequate sedation, and if there is any resistant at the posterior throat, the wire is pulled slightly while introducing the catheter to allow easier passage. The endoscope is reinserted along the introducer catheter to verify the balloons are in the stomach, ideally following the greater curvature of the stomach and below the cardia. Using an automatic inflation pump with saline and methylene blue, first the proximal and then the distal balloons are inflated under direct visualization. Each balloon catheter needs to be sealed with mineral oil (valve sealant) provided in the kit. The endoscope tip is positioned above the proximal balloon and both are withdrawn together against the gastroesophageal junction all the way out of the mouth. Then the patient is re-scoped for final inspection.

J. Ponce (✉)
Medical Director of Bariatric Surgery, CHI Memorial Hospital, Chattanooga, TN, USA

© Springer Nature Switzerland AG 2020
M. Galvao Neto et al. (eds.), *Intragastric Balloon for Weight Management*,
https://doi.org/10.1007/978-3-030-27897-7_10

Fig. 10.1 Saline-filled
dual intragastric balloon

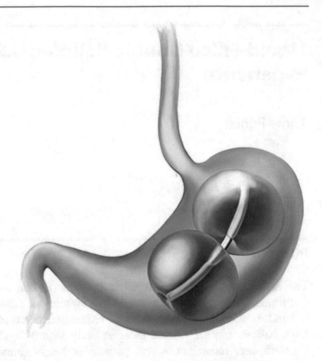

For removal, the scope is introduced. A suction puncture catheter is used to per-forate each balloon in perpendicular fashion and aspirate all fluid connecting it to suction. When aspiration is completed, the suction catheter is removed. A large endoscopic snare is used to securely grasp the proximal end cap around. Sometimes the end cap is difficult to see well and manipulation of the balloon with a grasper can allow easier view. Other option is to flip the device to allow the proximal cap to be at the distal end and use the scope in a retroflexion position to allow for easier visualization. While maintaining firm grasp, the scope is withdrawn while holding the snare together to remove the balloon and scope at the same time. After the device is out, the patient is re-scoped to do a final inspection (Fig. 10.2).

Patient Management

Patients always need to be instructed that before each endoscopy, they need to stay on clear liquids for 24 hours to avoid the presence of residual food in the stomach. This is especially important during the removal procedure. If food is present in the stomach, the endoscopic removal can be postponed, or the patient should be endo-tracheally intubated to protect the airway from bronchial aspiration of food particles.

Setting expectations is critical to avoid unexpected intense symptoms that could lead to the patient's request for early device removal. Patients with fluid-filled bal-loons should be advised that a certain level of nausea, vomiting, and abdominal pain

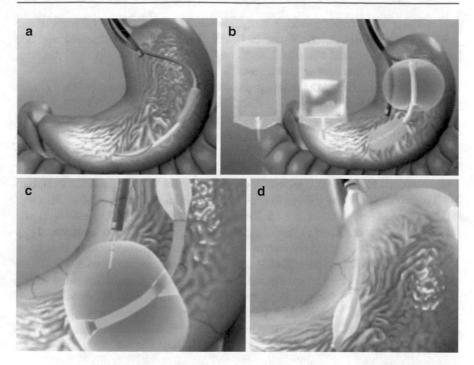

Fig. 10.2 Dual balloon placement and removal technique: (**a**) Place uninflated balloons; (**b**) Inflate proximal and distal balloon; (**c**) Puncture and aspirate balloons; (**d**) Remove with loop snare

can be expected for few days after balloon placement. A list of medications including analgesics, antiemetics, anxiolytics, and antispasmodics should be used. Patients will remain on clear liquids until significant nausea and/or vomiting subsides. Diet is usually progressed to solids over the first 1–2 weeks, and patients are educated to eat three small meals a day, small portions, chewing well each bite, eat a balanced diet, and avoid drinking liquids with high caloric content.

After balloon insertion, patients return to the clinic monthly for 6 months for medical supervision from an experienced bariatric multidisciplinary team. During these regular appointments, the integrated health team supports the patients in adhering to the weight loss program. They help patients develop healthy weight management skills, set goals, and monitor the patients' progress.

US Outcomes

US Food and Drug Administration (FDA) Clinical Study

The FDA approved the dual balloon on July 28, 2015, based on the REDUCE Pivotal Trial [1]. This study was a prospective, sham-controlled, double-blind, and randomized multicenter US clinical study that enrolled 326 patients with obesity and followed them for 48 weeks. Participants were between 21 and 60 years of age with a baseline BMI between 30 and 40 kg/m². Participants also presented with one or more obesity-related comorbid conditions, including type 2 diabetes mellitus, obstructive sleep apnea, or hypertension.

Patients were randomized into two groups. The treatment group ($n = 187$) had a balloon plus diet and exercise counseling. The control group ($n = 139$) underwent sham endoscopy plus diet and exercise alone. Balloon patients had the device removed after 24 weeks and continued with diet and exercise counseling for an additional 24 weeks. Balloon patients had a 28% excess weight loss (%EWL) or 7.6% total body weight loss (TBWL) at 24 weeks and 2.3 times as much weight loss compared to the control group. Twenty-four weeks after balloon removal, balloon patients maintained a mean of 66% of their initial weight loss. More than half of the subjects still had more than 25%EWL compared to baseline weight, and 25% of subjects continued to lose additional weight following device removal [1].

Adverse events included postimplantation accommodative symptoms of nausea, vomiting, and abdominal pain. Eighty-seven percent had nausea or vomiting. These symptoms were reported as mostly mild in severity and typically subsided within 3–7 days (Fig. 10.3). Early balloon removals were 15% with filling volumes of 900 mL and reduced to 7.7% when filling volumes were adjusted to height (750 mL on patients shorter than 64 inches). There was an incidence of 10% gastric ulcerations, the majority superficial, small at the level of the incisura.

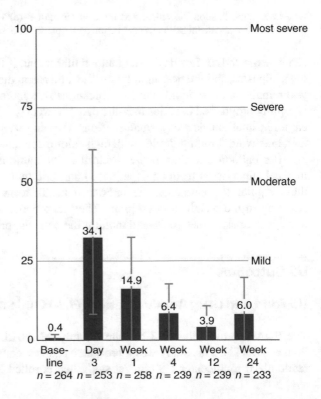

Fig. 10.3 Nausea and vomiting evaluated during the Reduce pivotal study [1]

Table 10.1 Dual balloon US studies outcomes

Device	Study type	Weight loss (6 months)	Early removal
Reshape [1]	RCT, multicenter, sham-controlled, double- blinded	7.6% TBWL 27.9%EWL	15% (900 mL) 7.7% (750 mL, height < 64"; 900 mL, height ≥ 64")
Morton [2]	Retrospective, multicenter	32.5%EWL	1%
Curry [3]	Retrospective, single center, comparative	10%TBWL	7.8%
Bennett [4]	Retrospective, single center, comparative	10.5%TBWL	7.7%

RCT Randomized Controlled Trial, TBWL Total Body Weight Loss, EWL Excess Weight Loss

Clinical US Experience After FDA Approval

There have been several reports of early experience with the dual intragastric balloon in clinical setting in the US. Morton et al. [2] reported experience in four US centers with 137 patients showing 32.5%EWL in average at 6 months and small incidence of complications including only one early balloon removal and 2% small gastric ulcers. Curry and Pitt [3] reported comparative experience in 100 patients with 10%TBWL with the dual balloon in 6 months and lower incidence of nausea and early removals compared to a single fluid-filled balloon. Same finding was shown by Bennett et al. [4] in a smaller comparative group where weight loss for the dual balloon group was 10.5%TBWL and early removals were half compared to the single fluid-filled balloon (Table 10.1).

Conclusion

Studies have shown that intragastric saline-filled dual balloon systems are an effective means of weight loss in patients suffering from obesity with BMI 30–40 kg/m² compared to diet and exercise management alone. Risk factors and limitations of the device include poor weight loss in up to 25–40% of the patients, nausea and vomiting in 60–90%, and intolerance requiring early removal in 1–15%. Considering that there is a significant number of people suffering from obesity that have tried multiple nonsurgical methods to lose weight, and the majority are still not ready or afraid to undergo a surgical intervention, the dual balloons are an effective and welcome addition to the bariatric surgeon's armamentarium for obesity treatment.

References

1. Ponce J, Woodman G, Swain J, et al. The REDUCE pivotal trial: a prospective randomized controlled pivotal trial of a dual intragastric balloon for the treatment of obesity. Surg Obes Relat Dis. 2015;11:874–81.

2. Morton J, Curry T, Nguyen N, Ponce J. Early experience with intragastric dual balloon as treatment for obesity. Surg Obes Relat Dis. 2016;12:S27.
3. Curry T, Pitt T. Intragastric balloon intolerance: a retrospective review of 100 patients treated with two different devices. Gastrointest Endosc. 2017;85:AB277–8.
4. Bennett MC, Early DS, Sullivan SA, et al. Comparison of two intragastric balloon systems for weight loss in a clinical setting. Gastrointest Endosc. 2017;85:AB280.

Mexican Experience in the Treatment of Obesity with Liquid-Filled Balloon

Martín Edgardo Rojano-Rodríguez, Enrique Rentería-Palomo,
Aida Monserrat Reséndiz-Barragán,
Guadalupe de los Ángeles Salinas-Cornejo,
and Luz Sujey Romero-Loera

Introduction

According to the National Health and Nutrition Survey of 2016, Mexico is facing a public health issue regarding obesity and overweight. The prevalence of both combined is 33.2% in children, 36.3% in teenagers, and 72.5% in adults (in 2016) [1–3].

The Garren–Edwards Bubble was the first endoscopic device used for the treatment of obesity, approved by the FDA in 1984, although it was removed from the market 4 years later due to the multiple complications associated with its use. Many devices have been developed since. Currently there are three FDA-approved devices in the United States for the treatment of obesity: Orbera® (Apollo Endosurgery, Inc., Austin, TX, USA), ReShape® Duo (ReShape Medical Inc., San Clemente, CA, USA), and Obalon® (Obalon Therapeutics Inc., Carlsbad, CA, USA), others being in the process of approval. A wider range of devices is found in Europe, such as Spatz® (Spatz Medical, Great Neck, NY, USA) and the Heliosphere BAG® (Helioscopie Medical Implants, Vienne, France) [4].

M. E. Rojano-Rodríguez (✉) · A. M. Reséndiz-Barragán · L. S. Romero-Loera
Department of Endoscopic Surgery, Minimally Invasive Gastrointestinal and Bariatric Surgery, Hospital Dr. Manuel Gea González, Mexico City, Mexico

E. Rentería-Palomo
Division of General and Endoscopic Surgery, Hospital Dr. Manuel Gea González, Mexico City, Mexico

G. de los Á. Salinas-Cornejo
Division of Clinical Nutrition, Hospital Dr. Manuel Gea González, Mexico City, Mexico

© Springer Nature Switzerland AG 2020
M. Galvao Neto et al. (eds.), *Intragastric Balloon for Weight Management*,
https://doi.org/10.1007/978-3-030-27897-7_11

Indications

In Mexico, the Health Department regulates the use of the intragastric balloon through guidelines that establish the following requirements: Patients must have a body mass index over 40 kg/m^2 (or 35 if comorbidities are associated), with a previous complete clinical and laboratory evaluation, and a multidisciplinary group that involves the psychology department, a clinical nutritionist, and the medical team appropriately certified for the insertion of the intragastric device. To meet these requirements, the Mexican College of Surgery for Obesity and Metabolic Diseases created, in collaboration with the pharmaceutical industry, the Clinical Guidelines of Psychology and Nutrition for the evaluation, management, and treatment of patients with intragastric balloon and gastric band. The same contraindications that are described in the international literature for the use of intragastric devices are ruled in Mexico, such as psychiatric disease, previous gastric surgery, intolerance to proton-pump inhibitors, hiatal hernia of 5 cm or greater, pregnancy, breastfeeding, among others [2, 3].

Nutritional Evaluation

In terms of nutrition, the preoperatory evaluation includes an anthropometric and biochemical evaluation with a complete medical history, emphasizing the alimentary aspects and lifestyle. The anthropometric assessment consists of taking measures of weight, size, body mass index, excess weight, fat excess weight, percentage of body fat, muscle mass, waist, abdominal and neck circumference, as well as a bioimpedance analysis. The biochemical evaluation, according to the Argentine consensus of nutrition in surgery of 2010, reviewed in 2014, consists of blood count with a count of platelets, blood sugar, kidney function tests, general urine test, and a lipid profile [5]. The assessment must be carefully done knowing the patient's condition and individualizing each case to determine if additional studies other than the usual are required. Dietary assessment evaluates the usual energy intake of the patient. Based on this, the reduction of energy intake is determined prior to any bariatric procedure. Since the patient tends to draw down to 50% of the caloric intake, it is important to know how their eating habits are. Having a balloon is different from person to person. Some find it a lot easier than others. The dietary guidelines include from day 1 to day 3 only liquids starting with simple water and if tolerated it is progressed to free fluids avoiding carbonated drinks, from day 4 to day 10 soft foods only, and beyond day 10 normal textured foods. The patient should have vitamin and mineral supplements for 6 months while they have the balloon [6].

Psychological Evaluation

The psychological intervention of the patient consists of three stages: the evaluation phase, the intervention phase, and the follow-up. In the evaluation phase, a structured interview is done, aimed at identifying the areas of opportunity that should be worked on, such as the presence of psychopathologies or dysfunctional eating patterns, the quality of the support network, the expectations and degree of motivation, among others. Also, a battery of tests is applied, oriented to provide support for the identification of anxiety and depression, binge eating, and affectations in the quality of life. The second phase is characterized by a cognitive-behavioral intervention aimed at modifying the maladaptive behavior of the patient and developing new skills that allow weight loss. This intervention is carried out during the time that the patient has placed the intragastric balloon and can be administered monthly. Finally, once the balloon is removed, the patient is provided with a psychological follow-up aimed at maintaining the progress obtained from the treatment and, in some cases, continuing with the weight loss. This final phase may last about 6 months. The battery of tests must be provided at the end of the second and third phases as well to enhance the effectiveness of the treatment.

Results

In a prospective study held by the Obesity Clinic of the Dr. Manuel Gea González General Hospital, the use of intragastric balloon was compared with a hypocaloric diet as a treatment for obesity. Forty-seven obese patients were chosen, 20 of them were treated with a hypocaloric diet while 27 patients were treated with an intragastric balloon. In the hypocaloric diet group, the average initial body weight was 115.91 kg with an initial BMI of 41.05 kg/m^2 and the average final body weight was 101.9 kg, the final BMI of 39.09 kg/m^2, with a TBW loss of 13.85 kg and an EWL of 22.89%. In the intragastric balloon group, the average initial body weight was 107.44 kg with an initial BMI 39.67 kg/m^2 and the average final weight was 99.34 kg with the final BMI 36.64 kg/m^2, with a TBW loss of 8.11 kg and an EWL of 13.46%. Independent variables were compared using the t-student test without a significant difference found. In conclusion, the intragastric balloon was found as an effective therapy when compared to a supervised hypocaloric diet [7].

A second study in the same hospital included 22 patients, 16 of whom were female and 6 were male, with an average age of 41.6 years (21–63), an average weight of 113.9 kg (68–250), and a mean BMI of 41.4 kg/m^2 (30–89). Out of the 22 patients, 15 presented with associated comorbidities, the Orbera® balloon was used in 17 patients and the Spatz® balloon was used in 5. Seven patients presented some degree of discomfort after the procedure, nausea being the most prevalent symptom ($n = 4$), followed by vomit ($n = 3$), diarrhea ($n = 2$), and abdominal pain and bloating in one patient. A higher %EWL was seen in the group of patients with Spatz® balloon compared with Orbera® group. A %EWL during the first 6 months of follow-up was of 34.9%, although a regain of 40% of weight was seen 6 months after retrieval [8].

Another retrospective study included 53 patients that did not meet the criteria for bariatric surgery and had BMI under 35 kg/m^2. The average age was 33 years (17–63), 14 male and 39 female patients were included, with an initial average weight of 86.1 kg (62.1–121.4), the filling volume in average was of 612 ml (400–500), the time of follow-up at 1, 3, 6, 9, and > 9 months showed an excess body weight loss of 21.9%, 34.1%, 34.5%, 30.5%, and 43.5% respectively [9].

The Orbera® company was first registered in Mexico with the name BIB and then changed to its actual name in 2014. Data provided by this company reveals that 18,000 devices have been applied to patients in our country. There are 215 registered physicians to install the Orbera® balloon in Mexico. The minimum body mass index authorized by COFEPRIS for the use of the Orbera balloon is of 27 kg/m^2.

Regarding the Spatz® balloon, the COFEPRIS authorized its use in February 2015. Since then, more than 16,000 devices have been applied in our country, and currently, more than 1600 devices are being installed every month. Mexico City, Monterrey, Tijuana, Ciudad Juarez, Nuevo Laredo, and Reynosa are the cities in which more Spatz® balloons are being installed both in the private and public sectors. The percentage of associated complications is of 0.7%, gastric ulcer is the most common one, and in the majority of cases, it is related to the lack of adherence to medical instructions.

Conclusions

There are two main indications for the use of an intragastric balloon in Mexico. The first one is a bridge therapy in patients with super obesity to improve their conditions before definitive surgical therapy. The second main indication is for patients that do not meet the criteria for surgery and have a body mass index between 27 and 35 kg/m^2; and in this group, the weight loss is efficiently controlled by a multidisciplinary group.

In Mexico, the insertion technique is dictated by guidelines established by the Health Department and the pharmaceutical industry based on national and international security standards.

The results observed until now with the use of an intragastric balloon in Mexican population are in accordance with the international literature; nevertheless, multicentric analysis and meta-analysis are needed to verify such findings. In conclusion, the best results depend greatly on the multidisciplinary approach given to patients that are candidates for the use of the intragastric balloon.

References

1. ENSANUT (2016) Encuesta Nacional de Salud y Nutrición de Medio Camino. 3–6.
2. Secretaria de salud (2010) NORMA Oficial Mexicana NOM-008-SSA3-2010, Para el tratamiento integral del sobrepeso y la obesidad. Cuidad de México.
3. CENETEC Consejo de Salubridad General (2012) Prevención, Diagnóstico y Tratamiento del Sobrepeso y la obesidad Exógena 15–21.
4. Gleysteen JJ. A history of intragastric balloons. Surg Obes Relat Dis. 2016;12(2):430–5.
5. Fantelli Pateiro L, Pampillon N, Coqueugniot M, De Rosa P, Pagano C, Reynoso C, et al. Nutritional graph for Argentina's bariatric population. Nutr Hosp. 2014;29(6):1305–10.

6. The Department of Nutrition and Dietetics St George's Hospital NHS Trust (2011) Your diet following intra-gastric balloon placement. 1–7.
7. Beristain Hernández J, Rojano Rodríguez M, Moreno Portillo M (2011) Comparación en el manejo de la obesidad entre el balón intragástrico y una dieta hipocalórica supervisada. XIII Congreso Nacional de Cirugía de la Obesidad y Enfermedades Metabólicas.
8. Topete L, Rojano Rodríguez M, Romero Loera L (2018) Determinar el porcentaje de exceso de peso perdido y reganancia de peso en pacientes con uso de balón intragástrico de la población de la Clínica de obesidad del Hospital General "Dr. Manuel Gea González" en los últimos 5 años. Ciudad de México.
9. García de Alba Nuñez, Rodríguez Huerta N, Jaramillo de la Torre E (2009) REPORTE DE RESULTADOS CON EL USO DEL BALÓN INTRAGÁSTRICO NO CANDIDATOS A CIRUGÍA BARIÁTRICA. XI Congreso Nacional de Cirugía de la Obesidad y Enfermedades Metabólicas.

Obalon Intragastric Balloon System Overview

12

Andre F. Teixeira, Muhammad Jawad, and Rena Moon

History

The use of gastric filling devices to induce weight loss is not new. Free-floating intragastric balloons were used by Nieben and Harboe in 1982 [1]. Percival presented a "balloon diet" in 1984 when he placed inflated mammary implants as gastric balloons [2]. In 1985, the Garren–Edwards Bubble was introduced as the first FDA-approved device, but the approval was withdrawn 7 years later because of complications [3]. Analysis of its problems led to recommendations for safer designs [4]. While a number of further developed devices were used outside of the United States, mostly in Europe and South America.

Introduction

A gastric balloon is an inflatable medical device that is temporarily placed into the stomach to reduce weight. It is marketed to provide weight loss when diet and exercise have failed, and surgery is not wanted or not recommended. Intragastric balloon therapy is a temporary method of inducing weight loss. It relies in a balloon placed in the stomach to promote the feeling of satiety and restriction. The weight loss mechanism is due to nature of causing restriction and the delaying gastric emptying.

Less intake of food will result in weight loss. After up to 6 months, the device is removed using endoscopy. Longer stay of a balloon is not advised because of the danger of damage to the tissue wall and degradation of the balloon. The use of the balloon is complemented with counseling and nutritional support or advice.

The indications for intragastric balloon therapy, the placement the adverse events, indication, and contraindications are discussed here in this chapter.

A. F. Teixeira (✉) · M. Jawad · R. Moon
Department of Bariatric Surgery, Orlando Health Institute, Orlando, FL, USA
e-mail: andre.teixeira@orlandohealth.com

© Springer Nature Switzerland AG 2020
M. Galvao Neto et al. (eds.), *Intragastric Balloon for Weight Management*,
https://doi.org/10.1007/978-3-030-27897-7_12

Obalon Balloon Inflation System Overview

The Obalon® Balloon System (Obalon Therapeutics Inc., Carlsbad, CA, USA) is designed to assist weight loss by partially filling the stomach. The system consists of up to three intragastric balloons placed during a 6-month period. The balloons are swallowable (Fig. 12.1), and each balloon is placed individually within the first 3 months. The removal is done endoscopically at the 6 months mark after the first balloon was placed.

Each balloon is contained within a porcine gelatin capsule, which is attached to a catheter. The balloon capsule delivers the balloon in a similar manner that a medicinal capsule delivers pharmaceuticals. The catheter comes pre-attached to the compacted balloon's radio-opaque, resealing valve.

The Obalon Balloons must only be inflated utilizing the EzFill Inflation System®. The EzFill® Inflation System consists of an EzFill® Can and EzFill® Dispenser. The can is intended to provide a gas source for transfer of a fixed volume of inflation gas to the Obalon® Balloon.

Obalon® Balloon US Pivotal Trial was the *Six-Month* Adjunctive Weight *Reduction Therapy* (SMART) Trial, where 336 patients showed no serious adverse events that were device or procedure related.

The conclusions of that trial were:

- Strong safety profile
- 0.3% serious-ADE rate of 1 in 336 subjects
- Progressive weight loss over full 6 months
- Statistically significant improvement in key metabolic parameters
- Strong weight loss maintenance
- 89.5% of mean TWL achieved at 6 months retained at 1 year

Fig. 12.1 Balloon capsule

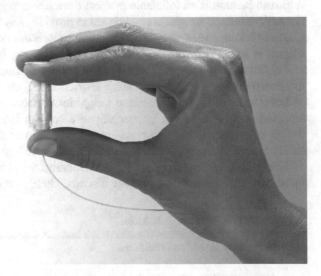

Placement

The EzFill® Inflation System is prepared prior to balloon administration away from the patient. The Extension Tube from the Accessory Kit is attached on the proximal end to the EzFill® Dispenser (Fig. 12.2) using a luer connection, while a three-way stopcock valve on the distal end of the Extension Tube remains closed. The green valve on the EzFill® Dispenser is turned to the on position and the EzFill® Can is inserted into the Dispenser. The lever on the Dispenser is closed to secure the Can in place and acts as a valve in the Can pressurizing the system; the Dispenser audibly releases excess pressure in the Can via its mechanical pressure relief system to ensure a starting pressure appropriate for the altitude at which the system is operated. The Dispenser contains a digital pressure gauge that provides a continuous read-out of the pressure inside the Can. Prior to initiating each step in the inflation process, the pressure gauge value is verified to ensure that it is stable for at least 30 seconds (not changing more than 0.3 kPa) at each decision point to ensure there are no leaks in the system.

After the capsule is swallowed, the EzFill® Inflation System is connected to the catheter by way of the extension tube. All entries and exits within the Dispenser and Catheter connections are sealed, and it is imperative that all system connections are fully secured during the procedure to maintain a closed gas pathway between the Can and Balloon.

The placement procedure is done at the radiology suite without any sedation. The catheter/capsule is swallowed by the patient, and by using the fluoroscopy system in the radiology suite, we can visualize the radio-opaque valve inside the stomach.

The catheter is then attached to the EzFill® Dispenser. EzFill® Can that contains nitrogen–sulfur hexafluoride gas mixture to fill the balloon is attached to the dispenser. Once there is radiographic confirmation that the balloon is below the gastroesophageal junction, the balloon is inflated. After inflation is complete, the catheter is ejected from the balloon valve and retrieved, leaving each balloon free-floating in the patient's stomach.

A fully inflated single balloon is an ellipsoid with a volume of approximately 250 cc. When three balloons are placed, the total balloon volume is approximately 750 cc. The balloons are only intended to remain in the stomach for 6 months from the time of placement of the first balloon. There should be no less than 14 days between each balloon placement. All balloons placed must be removed at the end

Fig. 12.2 Insufflator
device

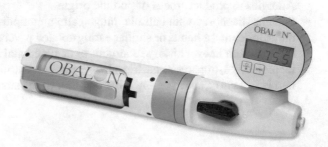

of 6 months after placement of the first balloon, using endoscopy per the specified tool dimensions. All placed balloons must be removed by a credentialed physician trained in endoscopy and foreign object retrieval.

Medications Post Placement

Proton-pump inhibitors should be prescribed for the duration of implantation. Antiemetic and antispasmodic medication are required at least 24 hours prior to administration and use for up to 5 days beyond balloon administration.

Indications for Use

The intragastric balloon system is indicated for temporary use to facilitate weight loss in adults with obesity (BMI of 30–40 kg/m^2) who have failed to lose weight through diet and exercise. The system is intended to be used as an adjunct to a moderate intensity diet and behavior modification program. All balloons must be removed 6 months after the first balloon is placed.

Contraindications

- Anatomical abnormalities or functional disorders that may inhibit swallowing or passage through any portion of the entire gastrointestinal (GI) Tract
- Prior surgeries that may have resulted in intestinal adhesions, narrowing of any portion of the digestive tract, or any other condition that may inhibit passage through any portion of the GI tract
- Persons who have undergone any bariatric surgery procedure
- Inflammatory and other pathophysiological conditions of the GI tract
- Chronic or acute use of medications known to be gastric irritants or to otherwise alter function or integrity of any portion of the GI tract, including but not limited to NSAIDs and aspirin
- Untreated *Helicobacter pylori* infection
- Patients who are unable or unwilling to take prescribed proton-pump inhibitor medication for the duration of the device implant
- Allergies to products/foods of porcine origin
- Patients diagnosed with bulimia, binge eating, compulsive overeating, high liquid calorie intake habits or similar eating-related psychological disorders
- Patients with known history of structural or functional disorders of the stomach including, gastroparesis, gastric ulcer, chronic gastritis, gastric varices, hiatal hernia (>2 cm), cancer, or any other disorder of the stomach

- Patients requiring the use of antiplatelet drugs or other agents affecting the normal clotting of blood.
- Pregnant or lactating women, or women with an intent to become pregnant
- Known history of duodenal ulcer, intestinal diverticula (diverticulitis), intestinal varices, intestinal stricture/stenosis, small bowel obstruction, or any other obstructive disorder of the gastrointestinal tract
- Known history of irritable bowel syndrome, radiation enteritis, or other inflammatory bowel disease, such as Crohn's disease
- Patients taking medications on specified hourly intervals that may be affected by changes in gastric emptying, such as antiseizure or antiarrhythmic medications
- Alcoholism or drug addiction

Adverse Reactions

The following patient complications associated with use of the Obalon Balloon System were noted in clinical studies:

Most frequently occurring events (>50%):
- Abdominal pain
- Nausea

Frequently occurring events (10–20%):
- Vomiting
- Indigestion/heartburn
- Bloating

Less frequently reported events (1–9.9%):
- Burping/belching
- Diarrhea
- Gastric irritation
- Gastric bleeding/abrasion
- Esophageal bleeding/abrasion
- Esophagogastric bleeding/abrasion
- Constipation
- Difficulty in sleeping
- Excessive gas
- Esophagitis
- Headache
- Oxygen desaturation

Rarely reported events include (<1%):
- Chest pain
- Gastric ulcer
- Hypersalivation
- Device intolerance
- Shortness of breath
- Sore throat
- Vocal cord spasm
- Allergic reaction
- Asthma
- Coughing
- Dizziness
- Dry heaving
- Fatigue
- Food passage difficulty
- Fullness
- Hiccups
- Hypertension
- Peptic ulcer disease
- Retaining food and fluid
- Shoulder pain
- Swollen lips
- Syncope
- Halitosis-bad breath

Extremely rarely reported events observed in global experience (<0.05%):
- Balloon deflation or migration that leads to a bowel obstruction requiring surgery to remove it

Less than 0.01%:
- Esophageal rupture requiring surgical repair (Europe)
- Esophageal rupture requiring surgical repair with resulting in sepsis and ultimately death (Mexico)

Possible complications resulting from balloon therapy that have not been reported in the US study or globally to date include:
- Perforation or rupture of the stomach

Additional complications that can be associated with endoscopy include:
- Abdominal cramps or discomfort from the air used to distend the stomach
- Allergic or adverse reaction to sedation or anesthesia
- Aspiration (of liquid or food if present in stomach during balloon removal procedure)
- Cardiac or respiratory arrest (these are extremely rare and are usually related to severe underlying medical problems)

- Digestive tract injury or perforation
- Sore or irritated throat following the procedure
- Excessive sweating
- Hypotension
- Impaired judgment or reactions after sedation or anesthesia
- Laryngospasm

Conclusions

The Obalon® Balloon System is an air-filled balloon designed to assist weight loss by partially filling the stomach. The system consists of up to three intragastric balloons placed during a 6-month period. Weight loss results are satisfactory, with a good safety profile.

References

1. Neiben OG, Harboe H. Intragastric balloon as an artificial bezoar for treatment of obesity. Lancet. 1982:198–9. https://doi.org/10.1016/s0140-6736(82)90762-0.
2. Percival WL. The balloon diet: non-invasive treatment invasive treatment for morbid obesity: preliminary report on 108 patients. Can J Surg. 1984;27:135–6.
3. Gleysteen JJ. A history of intragastric balloons. Surg Obes Relat Dis. 2016;12(2):430–5. https://doi.org/10.1016/j.soard.2015.10.074. PMID 26775045.
4. Gaur S, Levy S, Mathus-Vliegen L, Chuttani R. Balancing risk and reward: a critical review of the intragastric balloon for weight loss. Gastrointest Endos. 81:1330–6. https://doi.org/10.1016/j.gie.2015.01.054. PMID 25887720.

The US Experience with Swallowable Gas-Filled Balloons

13

Mark Gromski and Shelby Sullivan

The Obalon Balloon System (Obalon Therapeutics, Carlsbad, CA) is currently the only swallowable gas-filled balloon approved for use in the United States. The Obalon Balloon System was approved by the Food and Drug Administration (FDA) on September 8, 2016 [1], and the new placement system that does not require fluoroscopy or digital X-ray for placement (Obalon Navigation-Touch System) was approved by the FDA on December 20, 2018 (Fig. 13.1). Each balloon is delivered by swallowing a capsule containing the deflated balloon, which is attached to a thin (2 French) peroral catheter (Fig. 13.2). Once swallowed and with verification of the balloon in the stomach through the Navigation-Touch System, the Touch Dispenser delivers a nitrogen mixture of gas through the catheter to inflate the balloon to 250 mL (Figs. 13.2 and 13.3). Thus, delivery of the swallowable gas-filled balloon system does not require endoscopy or sedation. Three balloons are placed over a period of 6–12 weeks unless patients have non-resolved accommodative symptoms and remain in place for a 6-month treatment period. At the conclusion of the treatment period, the balloons are deflated and retrieved with standard endoscopic instruments. It is approved for use in patients with obesity with a body mass index (BMI) of 30–40 kg/m^2 who have failed to achieve sustained weight loss through diet and exercise.

The pivotal trial leading to the FDA approval of the device was recently published [2]. The trial was a double-blind, randomized, sham-controlled trial. Fifteen centers including both private practice and academic centers from the United States participated. Patients with a BMI of 30–40 kg/m^2 and aged 22–60 years were included in the study with 1:1 randomization to capsules containing balloons or capsules containing a sugar ribbon at weeks 0, 3, and either 9 or 12. All subjects

M. Gromski
Indiana University School of Medicine, Indianapolis, IN, USA

S. Sullivan (✉)
University of Colorado School of Medicine, Aurora, CO, USA
e-mail: SHELBY.SULLIVAN@CUANSCHUTZ.EDU

© Springer Nature Switzerland AG 2020
M. Galvao Neto et al. (eds.), *Intragastric Balloon for Weight Management*,
https://doi.org/10.1007/978-3-030-27897-7_13

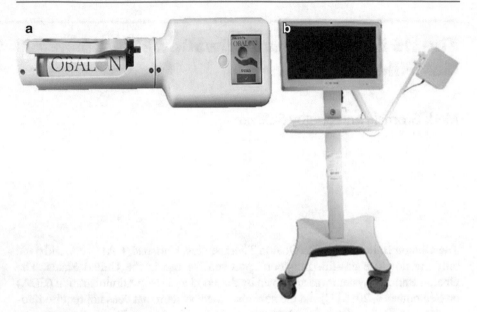

Fig. 13.1 Panel (**a**): Touch Dispenser. Panel (**b**): Navigation Console and field generator

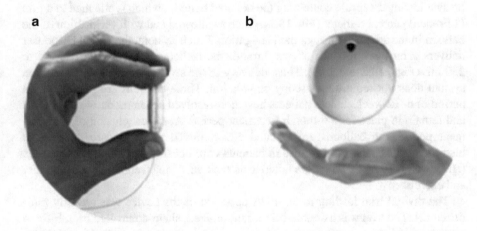

Fig. 13.2 Obalon Balloon System. Panel (**a**): Balloon inside capsule attached to inflation catheter. Panel (**b**): Balloon fully inflate (Reprinted with permission from Elsevier)

underwent moderate intensity lifestyle therapy with a registered dietitian every 3 weeks. All balloons were removed at week 24. A total of 387 patients swallowed at least 1 capsule. Of those patients, 93.3% of patients completed all 24 weeks of blinded study testing. For all patients who completed treatment, the treatment group (Obalon) achieved 7.1% TBWL, while the control (sham) achieved 3.6% TBWL ($p < 0.01$) [2]. The responder rate in the treatment group was 66.7% ($P < 0.0001$), and weight loss maintenance in the treatment group was 88.5% at

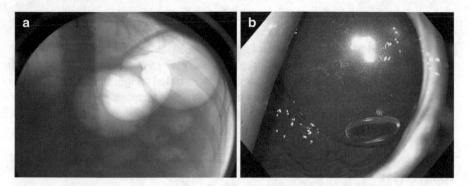

Fig. 13.3 Panel (**a**): Three Obalon Balloons in the stomach on Fluoroscopy. Panel (**b**): Endoscopic image of Obalon Balloons inflated in the stomach

48 weeks [2]. The average balloon administration and inflation time in the active group was 9.8 minutes. The three-balloon removal procedure time was 15.6 minutes and is performed by aspirating the gas out of the balloon with an injection needle connected to suction, followed by securing with a 15 mm or larger rat-toothed alligator forceps for extraction through the mouth with these steps repeated for the second and third balloons [2].

The treatment group had significant improvements in several cardiometabolic outcomes compared to the sham group, including decreases in systolic blood pressure, plasma total cholesterol concentration, plasma triglyceride concentration, and plasma glucose concentration [2].

No unanticipated device events occurred. There was 1 (0.3%) serious adverse event, which was a gastric ulcer in a patient taking protocol-prohibited nonsteroidal anti-inflammatory drugs. Nonserious adverse events occurred in 305 subjects, and 99.5% of adverse events were rated as mild or moderate. One balloon deflation occurred in the trial for a rate of 0.1%. Less than 3% of events related to the balloon required additional diagnostic procedure or intervention outside of prescription medications.

A prospective registry study containing 1343 patients receiving the swallowable gas-filled balloon system across 108 treating physicians was recently published [3]. This provides "real-world" clinical data with regard to the system. Intended use with three balloons for at least 20 weeks was achieved in 82.1% of patients. In this study, weight loss in the group of patients with a BMI of 30–40 kg/m^2 was 10.0% TBW. Weight loss for patients with a BMI of >40 kg/m^2 was 9.3% TBW and for patients with a BMI of 25–29.9 kg/m^2 was 10.3%.

In this study, there were seven balloon deflations (0.18%), none of which caused obstruction. Nonserious adverse events were reported in 14.2% of patients, and serious adverse events were reported in 0.15% of patients [3]. One of the serious adverse events reported was a cratered gastric ulcer with associated gastric perforation, in a patient who was not compliant with recommended proton pump inhibitor therapy. The most frequent nonserious adverse events were abdominal pain (5.3%), nausea (4.7%), vomiting (2.3%), and abdominal distention (1.0%) [3].

In summary, the randomized sham-controlled trial of the swallowable gas-filled balloon in the United States demonstrated twice as much weight loss in the balloon group compared with the sham control group and was safe with a low rate of serious adverse events. A large prospective registry study of over one thousand patients treated in the first year since FDA approval demonstrated weight loss efficacy superior to the randomized controlled trial and a low rate of adverse events. To date, no deaths have been reported from the swallowable gas-filled balloon system approved in the United States [4].

References

1. FDA. Summary of safety and effectiveness data (SSED) Obalon balloon system: FDA; 2016. p. 1–46.
2. Sullivan S, Swain J, Woodman G, et al. Randomized sham-controlled trial of the 6-month swallowable gas-filled intragastric balloon system for weight loss. Surg Obes Relat Dis. 2018;14(12):1876–89.
3. Moore RL, Seger MV, Garber SM, et al. Clinical safety and effectiveness of a swallowable gas-filled intragastric balloon system for weight loss: consecutively treated patients in the initial year of U.S. commercialization. Surg Obes Relat Dis. 2019;15(3):417–23.
4. Driscoll MDA letter to health care providers related to potential risks, including death, with liquid-filled intragastric balloons for weight loss NOT related to the Obalon gas-filled balloon. 2018. Accessed 6-7-18, 2018.

First Human Studies on Swallowable, Gas-Filled Balloon: The Obalon Balloon

14

Ariel Ortiz Lagardere

Introduction

Gastric balloons have been around since the latter part of the twentieth century [1]. Our experience with balloons started in the late 1990s when we were approached by Bioenterics (Carpinteria California), the company responsible for developing the BIB™ or Bioenterics Intragastric Balloon. At that time, we were involved in human trials of the balloon as well as evaluating safety and efficacy, but no randomized studies were available [2]. This device was approved for clinical use in Mexico and was used sporadically in our practice. The use of this specific balloon spread to other countries in America, including Brazil, where it was used extensively. In 2008, the authors were approached by a startup company supported by Domain, V.C. (Del Mar California), Obalon Therapeutics, out of Carlsbad California. A novel idea was introduced: A swallowable gastric balloon [3]. The authors agreed to participate in the clinical development and implementation of the device and registered several human studies in the Mexican Ministry of Health, COFEPRIS.

A. O. Lagardere (✉)
Obesity Control Center, Joint Commission Accredited, SRC, International Center of Excellence in Bariatric and Metabolic Surgery, CSG, Tijuana, Baja California, Mexico

University of Baja California, School of Medicine, Mexicali, Baja California, Mexico

University Ibero-Americana, School of Nursing Baja California, Tijuana, Baja California, Mexico

Obesity Control Center, Tijuana, Baja California, Mexico
e-mail: drortiz@obesitycontrolcenter.com

© Springer Nature Switzerland AG 2020
M. Galvao Neto et al. (eds.), *Intragastric Balloon for Weight Management*,
https://doi.org/10.1007/978-3-030-27897-7_14

Clinical Experience

Three studies were designed to focus on safe deployment and inflation of the device, tolerability, and endoscopic removal. The duration was 1, 2, and 3 months, respectively. During this phase of development, the protocol involved a preselected group of patients that were to undergo the procedure. Extensive information was given to the patient, consent forms were signed, and an initial medical assessment was performed by our internal medicine team. Blood samples for baselines were drawn, and patients were prepared with antiemetics and acid pump inhibitors before the procedure.

A total of 28 patients with a BMI of 34.8 were enrolled in three trials lasting 1, 2, and 3 months. Patients were monitored for tolerance to the balloon, complications, and weight loss (Slide 14.1).

Patients were asked to swallow the capsule attached to a miniature detachable catheter. Position of the balloon capsule was confirmed under fluoroscopy prior to inflation with gas (Slide 14.2).

The administration took less than 5 minutes. Only basic nutritional information was provided. Additional balloon placements were based on patient weight loss progress and reported satiety levels. There were no unexpected or serious adverse events, the balloons were well tolerated, and there were no requests for early removal (Slide 14.3).

The Obalon® Gastric Balloon produced consistent monthly weight loss in all three studies. Mean excess weight loss (EWL) at 1 month was 11.8+/− 9.7%, 13.8+/− 7.4%, and 16.9 +/− 22.7% with one 250 cc balloon in each of the three studies [4, 5].

Mean EWL was 23.9+/−16.4% and 25.8+/−31.5% for the studies with 2 months of treatment. The treatment with a second balloon added in the second month was

Slide 14.1 Overview of three studies

Study Evolution			
Study	Study Duration	Max Number of Balloons	Max Balloon Volume
1	1 Month	1	250cc
2	2 Months	2	500cc
3	3 Months	3	750cc

Slide 14.2 Obalon device
components

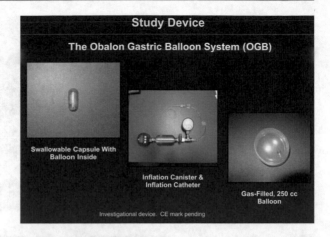

Slide 14.3 Adverse
events chart

Adverse Event	30 day (n=10)	60 day (n=8)	12 weeks (n=10)	All Studies (n=28)
Stomach cramps	9 (90%)	8 (100%)	0 (0%)	17 (60.7%)
Vomiting	6 (60%)	4 (4%)	1 (10%)	11 (39.3%)
Nausea	0 (0%)	3 (37.5%)	0 (0%)	3 (10.7%)
Diarrhea	0 (0%)	0 (0%)	1 (10%)	1 (3.5%)
Reflux	0 (0%)	2 (20%)	0 (0%)	2 (7.1%)
Ulcer (H. Pylori +)	3 (30%)	0 (0%)	0 (0%)	3 (10.7%)
Ulcer (H. Pylori -)	1 (10%)	0 (0%)	0 (0%)	1 (3.5%)
Esophageal laceration	3 (30%)	0 (0%)	0(0%)	3 (10.7%)

associated with greater weight loss as compared to the single balloon treatment. In the second study, five patients who received two balloons achieved a mean EWL of 35.9+/−36.9% (12.4–100/4%) at the end of 2 months. One subject lost 100% of her excess weight at the end of 2 months.

Patients in the final study had a mean EWL of 34.5+/−16.9% at the end of 3 months. All 10 patients were reviewed and received an additional balloon during the second month of treatment, and two patients received a third balloon in the third month (Slides 14.4, 14.5, 14.6, and 14.7).

The balloons were removed via endoscopy under light conscious sedation with procedures averaging less than 10 minutes per patients.

Conclusions of the three studies favor tolerability and safety from progressively utilizing up to three swallowable 250 cc gastric balloons, producing consistent weight loss and encouraging metabolic improvement. The ability to easily add balloon volume during the treatment period appears to improve treatment, weight loss, and tolerability.

Slide 14.4 Excess weight loss chart

Excess Weight Loss (%)			
	1 Month	2 Months	3 Months
Study 1	11.8±9.7*	N/A	N/A
Study 2	16.9±22.7*	25.8±31.5*	N/A
Study 3	19.0±6.8*	26.5±14.1*	34.5±16.9*
		*P < 0.01	

Slide 14.5 Total weight loss in percentage of TBW

Total Weight Loss (%)			
	1 Month	2 Months	3 Months
Study 1	2.9±1.8*	N/A	N/A
Study 2	2.6±2.0*	4.4±2.5*	N/A
Study 3	4.6±1.7*	6.5±3.8*	8.4±4.5*
		*P < 0.01	

Slide 14.6 Total weight loss in kilograms

Total Weight Loss (kg)			
	1 Month	2 Months	3 Months
Study 1	3.0± 1.7*	N/A	N/A
Study 2	2.5± 1.7*	3.8± 1.9*	N/A
Study 3	4.24± 1.7*	6.2±3.5*	7.9±4.4*
		*P < 0.01	

Discussion

The device is a folded polymer balloon within a gel capsule, the size of a large vitamin pill. This capsule is tethered to a thin inflation tubing on one end and attached to an inflation device with a proprietary gas mixture contained in a sealed pressurized

Slide 14.7 BMI reduction chart

	Reduction in BMI		
	1 Month	**2 Months**	**3 Months**
Study 1	1.06 ±0.63*	N/A	N/A
Study 2	0.87± 0.63*	1.44± 0.73*	N/A
Study 3	1.54± 0.63*	2.21± 1.35*	2.86±1.6*

$*P < 0.01$

canister. The placement of the device basically consisted in giving the patient the pill and asking to swallow it with water where two out of three patients would need a second effort to swallow the device. It should be noted that difficulty in swallowing the capsule would lead to early activation of the gel capsule and the device would be considered useless. Several instances happened where the device was swallowed but then fluoroscope control would demonstrate that the capsule with the balloon were dislodged at the lower third of the esophagus. A unique way of pushing the balloon down was by asking patients to eat and swallow large pieces of banana that led to the distal progression of the device into the gastric lumen. Once the device was in the lumen, a short waiting time of around 5 minutes was taken before actuating the inflation device. A canister placed in a calibration device with a manometer was connected to the inflation tube, and a remeasured gas volume was deployed. Once the pressures reached a certain level, the inflation tube was then disconnected from the inflation circuit and then connected to a string with water where hydrostatic pressure was used to release the tip of the inflation tubing to the balloon itself.

The Obalon® Balloon is a gas-filled device that was in a large series of fluoroscopies would normally reside in the highest part of the stomach mid body or fundus, depending on the number of balloons. A total of three balloons usually takes up the whole gastric fundus. Though the balloons are made of a light material and air-filled, the presence of these balloons without the use of acid blockers caused superficial ulcers and pain in one patient. This was resolved by reestablishing the acid blocking therapy on subsequent cases. During our clinical experience, we found that the biggest challenge was the swallowing of the device. We believe that this was a combination of the size of the capsule as well as the presence of the inflation tube that disrupts the normal pattern of swallowing. Several devices stopped their progression at the distal esophagus where the "banana technique" was used successfully. The most remarkable sensation reported by patients was feeling satiated immediately after inflation. This sensation was reported by over two-thirds of the cases.

All patients were placed on a special nutrition program, which included a liquid phase, a soft food phase, and a transition to normal consistency within 4 days after placing each balloon. Initially, the nutritional plan had an intermediate phase of soft foods, but symptoms related to pain, discomfort, or acid reflux subsided once in solid foods, thus, this phase was eliminated. The diet consisted of a very low-calorie diet (VLCD) of 800 kcal with a distribution of 35% protein, 30% fat, and 35% carbohydrates in five meals per day. As early satiety was expected, patients were asked to eat in a specific order: They had to eat protein first followed by vegetables and fruit, leaving grains, legumes, and flours to be eaten last; each meal included one to two servings of fats. Patients were educated to distinguish between processed and whole-fresh food and were asked to avoid commercial prepackaged products and prefer organic produce and grass-fed animal sources. They were also educated about toxic load and strategies to avoid toxicants from food and personal hygiene products. Patients who referred symptoms related to heartburn were allowed to eat rice cakes freely. The nutritional plan included taking a specific bariatric glyphosate-free protein, multivitamin, and probiotics supplements. All patients had a smartphone app created at our center, which provided real-time monitoring of food and water intake, recipes, exercise, and symptoms. In addition, this app provided daily tips on dietary habits, mindfulness, using food as medicine, meal planning, sleep hygiene, physical activity, and exercise.

Final Considerations

In the never-ending battle against obesity and metabolic disease, the most useful asset is weight loss surgery. There is a huge gap between those patients who qualify for a surgical procedure and the vast majority of patients who do not qualify but still are considered overweight and have evident metabolic impairment. It is here where this nonsurgical, swallowable gas-filled balloon can prove to have the best clinical application. This particular balloon has now evolved with several major improvements, including a more resilient balloon material, a proprietary gas that prevents deflation of the device, new inflation device, a non-X-ray location device, and a smaller gel capsule. It has been our position that a device that can potentially produce satiety should be paired with the other two components essential to a successful and durable outcome. These components include patient education on specific macronutrients and body metabolism and the actual nourishment of the body itself. Our program consists of a smartphone app that addresses all the educational aspects and tracks the patient's well-being and progress. The other component is a nutritional line composed of protein shake, multivitamins, and probiotics aimed at gut health and restoration as well as lean mass sparing. We just understand that we are treating diseases where the cause is poorly understood, and first line of defense is a comprehensive approach to controlling and potentially reverting the disease.

References

1. Gleysteen JJ. A history of intragastric balloons. Surg Obes Relat Dis. 2016;12(2):430–5. https://doi.org/10.1016/j.soard.2015.10.074. Epub 2015 Oct 16.

2. Genco A, Cipriano M, Bacci V, Cuzzolaro M, Materia A, Raparelli L, Docimo C, Lorenzo M, Basso N. BioEnterics Intragastric Balloon (BIB): a short-term, double-blind, randomised, controlled, crossover study on weight reduction in morbidly obese patients. Int J Obes. 2006;30(1):129–33.
3. Mion F, Ibrahim M, Marjoux S, Ponchon T, Dugardeyn S, Roman S, Deviere J. Swallowable Obalon® gastric balloons as an aid for weight loss: a pilot feasibility study. Obes Surg. 2013;23(5):730–3. https://doi.org/10.1007/s11695-013-0927-x.
4. Ortiz Lagardere A, Martinez Gamboa A, So V, Miranda GM, Arrambide LS, Garcia CC. Weight loss and metabolic improvement using a swallowable, volume-titratable gastric balloon system. Tijuana. Abstract: IFSO, European Chapter, Barcelona.: Obesity Control Center; 2012.
5. Ortiz Lagardere A, Martinez Gamboa A, So V, Miranda GM, Miguel LS, Garcia CC. A less invasive gastric volume reduction with safe and effective titration. Tijuana. Abstract: IFSO, European Chapter, Barcelona.: Obesity Control Center; 2012.

Part III

Technical Procedures and Related Issues

Material: What Is the Minimum, the Desirable, and the Optimal

15

Luiz Henrique Mazzonetto Mestieri
and Flávio Hayato Ejima

Introduction

The use of intragastric balloons (IGB) is becoming more common each day as obesity and overweight increases worldwide. In a recent survey done in Brazil with expert endoscopists, it was estimated that there are over 40,000 balloons placed among these professionals [1].

As the IGB is supposed to be a minimally invasive procedure, the risk for the patient must remain low, thus, some minimum material is necessary to perform insertion and removal of IGBs with safety.

One must assume that the patient is already well selected and prepared, with an upper endoscopy (EGD) showing no contraindications for the device placement [2]. The procedure must be performed by a registered/specialized physician, in a prepared room/suite, with adequate patient ventilation support and cardiac monitoring, under conscious sedation or general anesthesia [1, 3, 4].

Intragastric Balloon Insertion

The insertion of most fluid-filled IGBs is done under endoscopic direct visualization, and a standard gastroscope is always needed for the procedure [5]. Exception has to be made for the Spatz3® balloon (Spatz Medical, Great Neck, NY, USA), that is inserted attached to the scope, and the Ellipse® (Allurion Technologies Inc.,

L. H. M. Mestieri (✉)
Endoscopy Unit, Mestieri Clinic, Salto, SP, Brazil
e-mail: drluiz@mestieri.com.br

F. H. Ejima
Department of Endoscopy, IHBDF – SES, Brasília, DF, Brazil

© Springer Nature Switzerland AG 2020
M. Galvao Neto et al. (eds.), *Intragastric Balloon for Weight Management*,
https://doi.org/10.1007/978-3-030-27897-7_15

Table 15.1 Material needed for balloon implant

Minimum material	Desirable material	Optimum material
Intragastric balloon	Methylene blue	Removal accessories
60 cc syringe luer-lock tip	Additional balloon	
Saline solution (1000 cc)		
Lubricant gel		

Natick, MA, USA) and Obalon® (Obalon Therapeutics Inc., Carlsbad, CA, USA), which are both swallowable, and need no gastroscope – but X-ray visualization – to be inserted [6, 7].

For the Orbera® (Apollo Endosurgery, Inc., Austin, TX, USA), Spatz3, Medicone, Bioflex, ReShape (ReShape Medical Inc., San Clemente, CA, USA) and Heliosphere® BAG (Helioscopie Medical Implants, Vienne, France) [8–13] balloons, a 60 cc syringe is recommended for insufflation. Orbera, Spatz3, Medicone, ReShape, and GFE balloons are filled with saline and a methylene blue solution, according to the manufacturer.

Note: In the USA, FDA did not approve methylene blue for Orbera. Heliosphere BAG is an air-filled balloon.

Besides the gastroscope, the physician must have enough lubricant gel and all the recommended material for an unexpected balloon removal. An additional balloon is also recommended, for any uneventful happening (Table 15.1).

Intragastric Balloon Removal

Upon balloon removal, one must read the balloon manufacturer's instructions and be specifically trained for this procedure. The removal of an intragastric balloon has to be done under optimal circumstances always, as we must assume the stomach is full and there is risk of bronchial aspiration.

The removal of intragastric balloons can be performed under conscious sedation or general anesthesia [1, 4, 6]. After performing the esophagogastroduodenoscopy (EGD), the intragastric balloon is generally punctured with a needle, has its contents aspired to a vacuum system through a catheter, and then it is grasped and removed, under direct visualization [6] (Table 15.2).

There are specific catheters with needles for balloon puncture and aspiration, sold by many manufacturers such as G-Flex® and Albyn Medical®.

After puncturing the balloon with the needle, the needle is removed from the catheter, and the catheter is connected to a vacuum system to aspire the balloon contents. Under direct visualization, the physician must be sure the balloon is completely deflated before its removal. Note: For the Heliosphere® BAG, more than one puncture is recommended, as there's no risk of fluid leaks from the balloon to the stomach. This step can be done under frontal view or in retroflex view [6].

After complete suction of all the balloon contents, grasping and removal takes place. The optimal situation occurs when the combined rat tooth alligator grasping forceps apprehends a three-fold angle of the empty balloon. With a constant

Table 15.2 Material needed for balloon removal

Minimum material	Desirable material	Optimum material
Suction catheter with puncture needle	Foreign body combined rat tooth and alligator jaw forceps	Double Channel gastroscope
Balloon grasping forceps	Large diameter symmetrical or asymmetrical polypectomy snare	Gastric overtube
Lubricant gel	Cooking vegetable oil	McGill forceps
Vacuum system		Endoscopic scissors

traction, the balloon is brought to the gastroesophageal junction and pulled through the esophagus.

When the balloon reaches the upper esophageal sphincter, constant traction is maintained, and small deflation of the endotracheal tube might help balloon removal through the upper esophageal sphincter (UES) if the patient is under general anesthesia. In some cases, the grasping forceps tears the balloon or loses it, specifically when going through the lower esophageal sphincter (LES). For those situations, a large polypectomy snare may be useful, as it captures more of the balloon silicone.

For easier removals, hyoscine is used when the balloon reaches the lower esophageal sphincter, to avoid or diminish esophageal spasms [6]. Another very useful tool is canola oil. After balloon emptying, using the drainage catheter, 10–15 cc of vegetable cooking oil are sprayed over the distal esophagus, from the LES toward the mouth [14]. The balloon is then apprehended with the forceps or the snare and brought, with constant traction, to the mouth. The oil smooths the passage of the balloon through the esophagus.

A gastric overtube might be used if the LES is under constant spasm. After grasping the balloon in the stomach, the balloon is brought to the distal part of the overtube and then removed along with it. In some more difficult cases, the balloon valve offers a resistance during balloon removal. The use of endoscopic scissors is useful to cut the valve of the balloon, and the two parts are then removed separately.

Also, another useful method to remove the intragastric balloon is to use a double-channel therapeutic gastroscope. In one channel a grasping forceps is inserted, and at the other a polypectomy snare. Once inside the stomach, open the snare completely and advance the forceps through it, closing the snare around the forceps. Grasp the balloon with the forceps, bring balloon toward the scope and open the snare, closing it around the balloon, thus apprehending the balloon with two instruments. This method gives a secure way to retrieve the balloon [15, 16].

Conclusions

Insertion and removal of intragastric balloons is a safe, feasible, and reproducible procedure, as the minimum material is present in many endoscopy suites and adequate training for the physician is easily available.

Ideally, the performing physician must have all the optimum material available, if any complication occurs, decreasing the risks for the patient.

References

1. Neto MG, Silva LB, Grecco E, et al. Brazilian Intragastric Balloon Consensus Statement (BIBC): practical guidelines based on experience of over 40,000 cases. Surg Obes Relat Dis. 2017; https://doi.org/10.1016/j.soard.2017.09.528.
2. Sallet JA, Marchesini JB, Paiva DS, Komoto K, Pizani CE, Ribeiro MLB, Miguel P, Ferraz AM, Sallet PC. Brazilian multicenter study of the intragastric balloon. Obes Surg. 2004;14:991–8.
3. Coskun H, Aksakal C. Experience with sedation technique for intragastric balloon placement and removal [3]. Obes Surg. 2007;17:995–6.
4. Messina T, Genco A, Favaro R, Maselli R, Torchia F, Guidi F, Razza R, Aloi N, Piattelli M, Lorenzo M. Intragastric balloon positioning and removal: sedation or general anesthesia? Surg Endosc Other Interv Tech. 2011;25:3811–4.
5. Papademetriou M, Popov V. Intragastric balloons in clinical practice. Gastrointest Endosc Clin N Am. 2017;27:245–56.
6. Wahlen CH, Bastens B, Herve J, Malmendier C, Dallemagne B, Jehaes C, Markiewicz S, Monami B, Weerts J. The BioEnterics intragastric balloon (BIB): how to use it. Obes Surg. 2001;11:524–7.
7. (2018) Obalon. http://www.obalon.com/. Accessed 14 Jan 2018.
8. (2018) Orbera. https://www.orbera.com/for-hcp. Accessed 14 Jan 2018.
9. (2018) Spatz3. http://spatzmedical.com/doctors-area-login/. Accessed 13 Jan 2018.
10. (2018) Balão Corporea. https://www.balaocorporea.com.br. Accessed 15 Jan 2018.
11. (2018) Bioflex balão intragastrico. https://gfedobrasil.com.br/portfolio_item/bioflex-balao-intragastrico/. Accessed 9 Jan 2018.
12. (2018) ReShape. https://pro.reshapeready.com. Accessed 15 Jan 2018.
13. (2018) Heliosphere BAG. http://www.helioscopie.fr/en/heliosphere-bag.html. Accessed 13 Jan 2018.
14. Neto G, Campos J, Ferraz A, Dib R, Ferreira F, Moon R, Teixeira A. An alternative approach to intragastric balloon retrieval. Endoscopy. 2016;48:E73.
15. Jenkins JT, Galloway DJ. A simple novel technique for intragastric balloon retrieval. Obes Surg. 2005;15:122–4.
16. Galloro G, Sivero L, Magno L, Diamantis G, Pastore A, Karagiannopulos P, Inzirillo M, Formisano C, Iovino P. New technique for endoscopic removal of intragastric balloon placed for treatment of morbid obesity. Obes Surg. 2007;17:658–62.

Liquid-Filled Intragastric Balloon: Implant and Removal Techniques

16

Jimi Izaques Bifi Scarparo, Manoel Galvao Neto, and João Caetano Dallegrave Marchesini

Introduction

Intragastric balloon implant and removal, when performed by qualified specialists, are considered of easy technical performance. However, both of them have potential and serious complications if not carried out with caution [1–4].

The first step in safety is the adequate selection of patients, taking into account indications, contraindications, and specific preparation, following the protocol of each medical service or of the medical society of each country [2, 5]. In 2016, the first Brazilian Intragastric Balloon Consensus meeting was carried out and published, which may serve as a guideline of indications and contraindications for IGB procedures [6].

After adequate selection has been made, the balloon implant may be carried out as an outpatient procedure, usually lasting less than an hour. Conscious sedation performed by the endoscopist or general anesthesia performed by an anesthesiologist can be chosen, depending on the patient status and preference of the physician [7]. In the beginning of the learning curve, it is recommended to start with the maximum possible safety, with general anesthesia, and support of an anesthesiologist,

J. I. B. Scarparo (✉)
Department of Endoscopy, Ipiranga Hospital and Scarparo Scopia Clinic, São Paulo, SP, Brazil
e-mail: drjimi@scarparoscopia.com

M. Galvao Neto
Department Digestive Surgery, ABC Faculty of Medicine, São Paulo, SP, Brazil

Department of Bariatric Endoscopy, Endovitta Institute, São Paulo, SP, Brazil

J. C. D. Marchesini
Department of Surgery, Marcelino Champagnat Hospital, Curitiba, PR, Brazil

Former President, Brazilian Society for Bariatric and Metabolic Surgery, São Paulo, SP, Brazil

Department of Endoscopy, Mario Covas Medical School, São Paulo, SP, Brazil

© Springer Nature Switzerland AG 2020
M. Galvao Neto et al. (eds.), *Intragastric Balloon for Weight Management*,
https://doi.org/10.1007/978-3-030-27897-7_16

especially in the removal procedure, where the risk of bronchial aspiration is greater. Cardiac and respiratory monitoring are required, and basic life support and ventilation equipment should be available as well. The patient remains under observation for at least an hour after completion of the procedure.

Implant Technique

The steps for proper balloon implant are described:

Pre-procedure

1. A liquid diet is recommended for 3 days before the procedure. This tends to reduce the side effects after the procedure [6].
2. Fasting is required for at least 8 hours before the procedure.
3. Initiate a proton pump inhibitor (PPI) as soon as the decision for balloon implant is taken by the patient.

Procedure

1. Patient position: supine or left lateral decubitus [6, 8, 9].
2. Xylocaine spray in oropharynx as usual in any endoscopic procedure.
3. Proceed to intravenous sedation or general anesthesia (with previous planning and anesthesiologist support when preferred).
4. Endoscopic examination of esophagus, stomach, and duodenum, aspirating any gastric contents.
5. Removal of the endoscope.
6. If there are no organic or anatomical contraindications, proceed with the introduction of the empty balloon through the oropharynx, under direct view, as an orogastric tube (Fig. 16.1), until it reaches the stomach.

Fig. 16.1 External view of balloon introduction through oral cavity

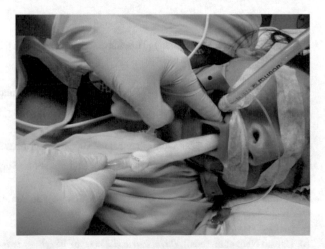

Fig. 16.2 Reinsertion of the endoscope, with care to keep the balloon in place

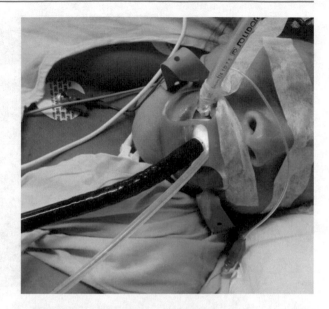

Fig. 16.3 Endoscopic view of IGB located in the gastric cavity, with enough space to expand

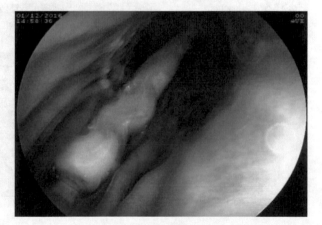

7. Reinsertion of the endoscope while keeping the balloon in place (Fig. 16.2), observing that the balloon has passed the lower esophageal sphincter and is well located within the gastric cavity (Fig. 16.3).
8. Removal of the guide wire from the balloon insertion tube (Fig. 16.4).
9. Connect the 60 (or 20) ml syringe to the two-way catheter.
10. Start inflating the balloon with the saline solution, with 10 ml of methylene blue added, if possible (this serves as a way of showing any leakage in the balloon) (Fig. 16.5) [6, 9].
11. Keep the stomach inflated with air to the maximum during filling, allowing the balloon to expand without resistance.
12. It is recommended to have a minimum of 500 ml inflated volume to avoid antral impaction, with a maximum of 700 ml.

Fig. 16.4 External view
of guidewire removed, to
start filling of the IGB

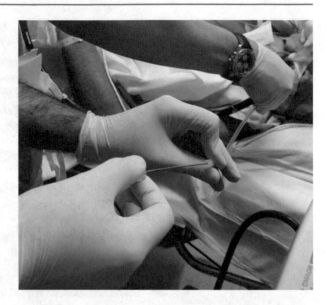

Fig. 16.5 Endoscopic
view of balloon filling

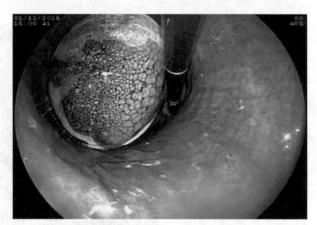

13. After the balloon is filled, proceed to release the balloon into the stomach.
    Make a suction of 50 ml of air, creating a vacuum and inverting the flow of the
    balloon valve, to avoid saline solution leaking. The valve of the balloon will be
    sealed by the vacuum created.
14. Smoothly start to pull the balloon against the cardia, in a cephalic traction of the
    inflation tube. This movement will disconnect the insertion tube from the bal-
    loon. This will happen when you feel a slight crack during the traction. After
    that, the balloon will be seen freely floating in the gastric cavity. It is necessary
    to slowly withdraw the tube and the outer wrapping of the balloon via the
    esophagus.
15. Proceed a review endoscopy of the balloon and its position. Ideal position is in
    the gastric fundus. Check if there is any kind of trauma of the stomach wall and
    esophagus.

16. All the maneuvers described in steps 7–14 should be preceded by direct endoscopic visualization.

After Procedure

1. The administration of the following drugs during or immediately after the implant procedure are recommended by the authors, decreasing post-implant symptoms: Omeprazol 20 mg – Dexamethasone 4 mg – Scopolamine 20 mg – Ondansetron 8 mg – Dimenhydrinate 100 mg – intravenously [6]. Eventually, Aprepitant 125 mg may also be used, to decrease nausea.
2. Keep a liquid diet for at least 10 days after the procedure, with regular follow-up with the dietitian after that.
3. Give comprehensive guidance to the patient and its family members about the side effects that may happen during the first few days.

Removal Technique

Before the Procedure

Differently from the balloon implant procedure, removal requires a lot of attention and preoperative care, due to the higher risk of complications during removal of the device.

After the balloon stay in the stomach, it is normal to have some gastroparesis, leading to food stasis, also due to the obstruction caused by the device. Thus, bronchial aspiration should be considered as the main complication during removal of the balloon. Some precautions are recommended before the procedure [8]:

1. The removal should be done preferentially under deep sedation done by an experienced endoscopist, or general anesthesia with orotracheal intubation, at the anesthesiologist's discretion, after cardiorespiratory assessment [8, 10].
2. It is recommended to drink sugar-free carbonated cola drinks, for at least 3 days prior to the procedure, in order to drain the content of food stasis in the stomach, decreasing the risk of bronchial aspiration.
3. Fasting of at least 10 hours is mandatory before the procedure.
4. The use of antiemetics drugs and bromopride is suggested, starting a week before the removal procedure, for the same purpose.
5. Avoid eating leafy vegetables and red meat a week before the procedure.

Procedure

1. After the patient is sedated, a digestive endoscopy is initiated. The endoscopist should go directly to the stomach and find the balloon (Fig. 16.6). Any gastric content should be aspirated, and the stomach is fully inflated.

Fig. 16.6 Removal procedure: endoscopic evaluation of balloon status

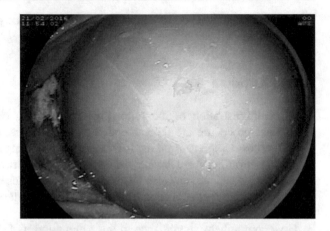

Fig. 16.7 Puncture of the balloon with proper needle for aspiration

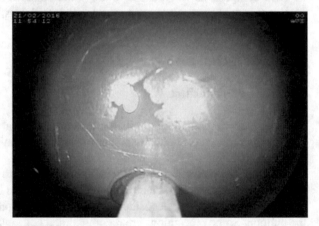

Puncturing of the balloon with frontal endoscopic view is done, using a proper needle (Fig. 16.7) [6, 9].

2. After puncture, the needle is penetrated some centimeters inside the balloon, usually at least 5 cm. The guidewire of the needle is removed, and aspiration is connected. A good aspiration device should be used, making aspiration as fast as possible. Suction of the liquid is initiated, measuring the aspirated volume if possible. The balloon needs to be completely empty in order to be removed (Fig. 16.8) [6, 9].

3. After the balloon is completely empty, using the same catheter is possible to smear lubricating oil in the whole esophagus. Cooking vegetable oil (10 ml) has been used with good results and no deleterious effects for the patient [11].

4. After that, the balloon is grabbed with the two-pronged wire grasper or, nowadays, with a large Raptor® (US Endoscopy, OH, USA) grasping device (a mixed rat-tooth and alligator grasper) (Fig. 16.9) [6]. The authors prefer to capture the empty balloon at the opposite end of the valve.

5. Initiate removal after intravenous injection of scopolamine 40 mg. Wait for tachycardia signs on the monitor and make a cephalic traction slowly. The

Fig. 16.8 Endoscopic view of balloon completely empty, ready for removal

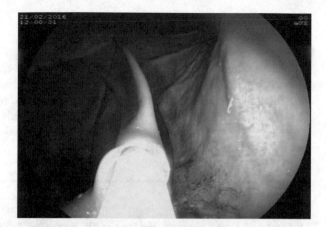

Fig. 16.9 Balloon removal with a Raptor® forceps

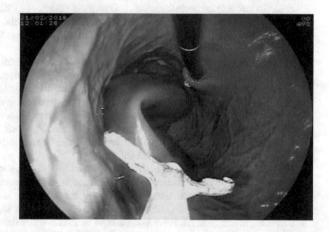

balloon should be extracted slowly and gradually. It should always be kept together with the tip of the endoscope, under direct view. The balloon passes through the cardia, esophagus, up to the oral cavity, and is extracted together with the endoscope.

6. Once the balloon is outside, an endoscopic revision is proceeded to check for any kind of complications, such as perforation, bleeding, trauma or laceration.
7. After removal, the patient should be kept under observation for at least 1 hour and then discharged.

After Procedure

1. It is recommended to take PPIs for 1 month after the procedure. Bromopride could be prescribed to help the stomach recover its usual peristalsis [6, 9].
2. The patient should keep a liquid diet for 3–5 days giving some rest to the organ.

Conclusions

The treatment with balloon has been growing worldwide, in our country more than 40,000 balloons have already been implanted. It is essential that new specialists are properly trained, increasing success of this procedure [10, 12, 13].

Although simple and safe, complications do exist and occur, with low incidence. These tend to be more frequent if the basic technical rules of implantation are not obeyed and the procedure is not performed by personnel who are properly trained and qualified to do so [12–14].

References

1. Force ABET, Committee AT, Abu Dayyeh BK, Edmundowicz SA, Jonnalagadda S, Kumar N, et al. Endoscopic bariatric therapies. Gastrointest Endosc. 2015;81(5):1073–86.
2. Gleysteen JJ. A history of intragastric balloons. Surg Obes Relat Dis. 2016;12(2):430–5.
3. Mathus-Vliegen EM. Intragastric balloon treatment for obesity: what does it really offer? Dig Dis. 2008;26(1):40–4.
4. Sallet JA, Marchesini JB, Paiva DS. The intragastric balloon. Endoluminal therapy for the treatment of obesity and metabolic disease. 3rd Edition – O Expresso – 2009. ISBN 85-8780624-6
5. Lopez-Nava G, Rubio MA, Prados S, Pastor G, Cruz MR, Companioni E, et al. BioEnterics(R) intragastric balloon (BIB(R)). Single ambulatory center Spanish experience with 714 consecutive patients treated with one or two consecutive balloons. Obes Surg. 2011;21(1):5–9.
6. Neto MG, Silva LB, Grecco E, de Quadros LG, Teixeira A, Souza T, et al. Brazilian Intragastric Balloon Consensus Statement (BIBC): practical guidelines based on experience of over 40,000 cases. Surg Obes Relat Dis. 2018;14(2):151–9.
7. Mitura K, Garnysz K. In search of the ideal patient for the intragastric balloon - short- and long-term results in 70 obese patients. Wideochir Inne Tech Maloinwazyjne. 2016;10(4):541–7.
8. Dai SC, Paley M, Chandrasekhara V. Intragastric balloons: an introduction and removal technique for the endoscopist. Gastrointest Endosc. 2015;82(6):1122.
9. Sallet JA, Marchesini JB, Paiva DS, Komoto K, Pizani CE, Ribeiro ML, et al. Brazilian multicenter study of the intragastric balloon. Obes Surg. 2004;14(7):991–8.
10. Imaz I, Martinez-Cervell C, Garcia-Alvarez EE, Sendra-Gutierrez JM, Gonzalez-Enriquez J. Safety and effectiveness of the intragastric balloon for obesity. A meta-analysis. Obes Surg. 2008;18(7):841–6.
11. Neto G, Campos J, Ferraz A, Dib R, Ferreira F, Moon R, et al. An alternative approach to intragastric balloon retrieval. Endoscopy. 2016;48(Suppl 1 UCTN):E73.
12. Gaur S, Levy S, Mathus-Vliegen L, Chuttani R. Balancing risk and reward: a critical review of the intragastric balloon for weight loss. Gastrointest Endosc. 2015;81(6):1330–6.
13. Force ABET, Committee AT, Abu Dayyeh BK, Kumar N, Edmundowicz SA, Jonnalagadda S, et al. ASGE Bariatric Endoscopy Task Force systematic review and meta-analysis assessing the ASGE PIVI thresholds for adopting endoscopic bariatric therapies. Gastrointest Endosc. 2015;82(3):425–38 e5.
14. Genco A, Lopez-Nava G, Wahlen C, Maselli R, Cipriano M, Sanchez MM, et al. Multi-Centre European experience with intragastric balloon in overweight populations: 13 years of experience. Obes Surg. 2013;23(4):515–21.

Adjustable Intragastric Balloon – Implantation and Removal

17

Ricardo José Fittipaldi-Fernandez, Eduardo N. Usuy Jr., João Antonio Schemberk Jr., and Vitor Ottoboni Brunaldi

Introduction

The adjustable intragastric balloon (Spatz®) is a water-filled device that may indwell for 1 year. Also, it has a specific catheter that allows volume adjustment at any time of the treatment. Some data already suggest that the adjustable balloon reduces significantly the early removal rate [1–3]. Therefore, it is an exciting device, but implantation and removal procedures have some particularities. The aim of this chapter is to describe the standard and alternative techniques to deploy and to retrieve the Spatz® balloon. Data on efficacy and safety are discussed elsewhere in this book.

Implantation of the Spatz® Balloon

As the nonadjustable balloon implantation, the first step of the procedure is an endoscopic examination of the upper digestive tract to exclude any contraindications for the balloon, such as esophageal rings, varices or strictures, large hiatal hernias, severe erosive esophagitis (Los Angeles grades C or D), neoplasia, or active peptic ulcers [4].

R. J. Fittipaldi-Fernandez (✉)
Department of Bariatric Endoscopy, Endogastro Rio Clinic, Rio de Janeiro, RJ, Brazil

E. N. Usuy Jr.
Department of Gastroenterology and Bariatric Endoscopy, Gástrica Clinic, Florianópolis, SC, Brazil
e-mail: usuy@usuy.com.br

J. A. Schemberk Jr.
Department of Endoscopy and Obesity, Obesogastro Clinic, Cutiriba, PR, Brazil

V. O. Brunaldi
Endoscopy Unit of the Department of Gastroenterology, (Hospital das Clínicas da Faculdade de Medicina da Universidade de São Paulo), University of São Paulo (Universidade de São Paulo), São Paulo, SP, Brazil
e-mail: vitor.brunaldi@usp.br

© Springer Nature Switzerland AG 2020
M. Galvao Neto et al. (eds.), *Intragastric Balloon for Weight Management*,
https://doi.org/10.1007/978-3-030-27897-7_17

Fig. 17.1 Balloon
attached to the scope

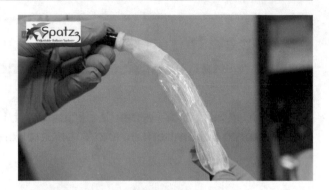

Fig. 17.2 Introduction
of the balloon

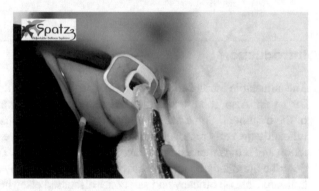

The standard technique, which is recommended by the manufacturer, is the introduction of the device side-to-side to the endoscope. In the balloon kit, there is a sleeve-like facilitator device that should be slid onto the extremity of the apparatus. The balloon should be placed alongside the endoscope with its tip parallel to the facilitator. The facilitator is then rolled back, thus embracing the distal edge of the balloon and attaching it to the endoscope (Fig. 17.1).

The whole arrangement is then generously lubricated with an appropriate gel, and the endoscope is gently and gradually introduced into the esophagus (Fig. 17.2).

Once the device reaches the gastric chamber, the endoscopist should perform a U-turn to ensure that the whole balloon is in the stomach and did not detach from the endoscope during the introduction. That maneuver avoids serious adverse events related to balloon-filling inside the esophagus (Fig. 17.3).

The balloon is then filled with 400 up to 700 ml of saline with methylene blue (in our daily practice, the standard volume is 600 ml). As the balloon fills up, it naturally detaches from the apparatus. Afterward, the endoscopist must pull the catheter used to fill the balloon until the valve appears in the patient's mouth (Fig. 17.4). During this step, we recommend the introduction of the forefinger into the patient's mouth to reach the base of the tongue and ensure that both catheter and valve slide smoothly, thereby avoiding any local scratches or bleeding. Then, the endoscopist should disconnect the catheter from the valve, and a special blue plug with a nylon loop on top should be attached to it (Fig. 17.5). This loop facilitates the reintroduction of the valve into the stomach using the endoscope.

Fig. 17.3 Checked
position of the balloon
inside the stomach

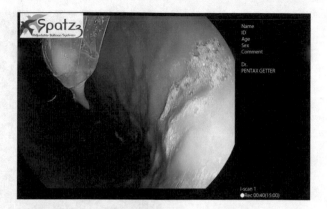

Fig. 17.4 Balloon valve

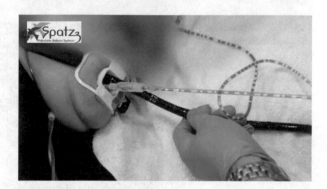

Fig. 17.5 Valve and nylon
loop

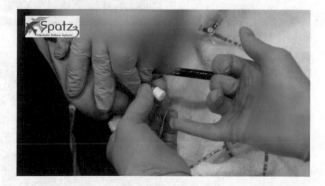

However, this technique is particularly challenging in short-necked patients. The large diameter of the device, when attached to the endoscope, may hinder the passage to the esophagus. Excessive pressure can cause laceration or perforation and should therefore be avoided.

To overcome that limitation, we developed a guided implantation technique. After the initial endoscopic examination, a metallic guidewire is placed in the antrum (Fig. 17.6). The endoscope is then withdrawn, and the balloon is attached to the plastic tube with an adhesive tape (Fig. 17.7). The device is introduced over the

Fig. 17.6 Metalic guide
wire introduction

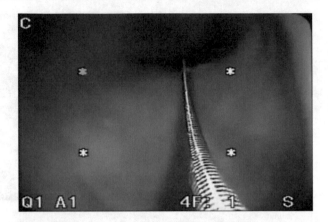

Fig. 17.7 Balloon is
attached to the plastic tube

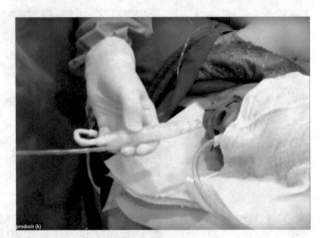

Fig. 17.8 Balloon being
filled under direct scope
view

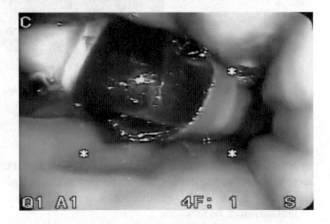

guidewire and positioned inside the stomach. Again, the apparatus must be inserted
to check the balloon's position. Under endoscopic control, the balloon should be
filled up (Fig. 17.8). Once filling is done, both wire and plastic tube should be withdrawn together. The remaining steps are similar to the standard implantation

technique. This alternative technique may reduce the risk of esophageal injury as the balloon does not pass simultaneously with the endoscope.

Balloon Adjustment Procedure

An upper endoscopy should be carried out after a liquid diet for 3–7 days plus 15 hours of fasting to avoid food residues in the stomach. With the patient under sedation, the endoscopist uses a foreign body forceps to grasp the nylon loop on the valve cap and retrieve it through the mouth. The protective cap must be unscrewed and the same catheter used to fill the balloon should be attached to the valve. The content is then aspirated or increased using a 60 cc syringe. Finally, the valve is disconnected, and the cap screwed back so it can be pulled back into the gastric chamber, similar to the implantation procedure.

Removal of the Balloon

Exactly as the adjustment procedure, the first step is an upper endoscopy after a liquid diet for 3–7 days plus 15 hours of fasting to avoid food residues. This strict recommendation is necessary since the balloon significantly impairs gastric emptying. Orotracheal intubation is currently controversial.

Two extremely experienced Brazilian groups advocate for or against the routine orotracheal intubation for the removal procedure.

The first group recommends intubation aiming at protection from any possible aspiration. The other group argues that some patients may have food residues in the stomach due to failure to adhere to the liquid diet, diabetic gastroparesis, or senile gastroparesis. Therefore, the intubation in any of those situations is risky by itself. The latter group recommends the procedure to be suspended in case of inadequate pre-procedural diet. Groups with a large experience with this approach have documented over 2500 removals without any report of endobronchial aspiration [5].

In our unit, the removal of the balloon has always been carried out without orotracheal intubation. However, we recommend routine orotracheal intubation for less-experienced teams.

There are two main techniques to deflate the balloon. The first method is similar to the adjustment procedure: the valve must be retrieved and brought out through the mouth of the patient. Then, the adjustment catheter is connected to it and used to deflate the balloon. We recommend such technique because it is practical and safe.

The alternative is by a puncture with an appropriate needle connected to a long catheter that should be attached to the aspiration, just as the standard balloon deflation.

Once the balloon is completely empty, it should be grasped using a grasper or polypectomy snare to capture the "tail," preferably at loop or the base where it is firm and less susceptible to rupture (Fig. 17.9). Then, scopolamine should be

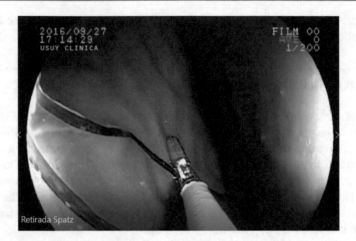

Fig. 17.9 An endoscopic grasper to the nylon loop

administered. The removal begins by applying a constant smooth traction. Once the endoscopist feels the balloon has overcome the resistance of the esophageal sphincter, the balloon usually slides out easily through the mouth of the patient.

Conclusion

The adjustable water-filled intragastric balloon (Spatz®) is an exciting device, but implantation, adjustment, and removal procedures have some peculiarities. The endoscopist must be aware of the standard technique and alternative ones to overcome any potential troublesome situation that may arise during the treatment with the Spatz balloon.

References

1. Evzen Machytka, Jeffrey Brooks, Marek Buzga, John Mason. One year adjustable intragastric balloon: safety and efficacy of the Spatz3 adjustable balloons. F1000 Research. 2014;Ago 3:203.
2. Brooks J, Srivastava ED, Mathus-Vliegen EM. One-year adjustable intragastric balloons: results in 73 consecutive patients in the U. K Obes Surg. 2014;24(5):813–9. https://doi.org/10.1007/s11695-014-1176-3.
3. Machytka E, Marinos G, Kerdahi RF, Srivastava ED, AlLehibi A, Mason J, Buzga M, Brooks J. Spatz Adjustable Balloons: results of adjustment for intolerance and for weight loss plateau. Gastroenterology. 2015;148(4, Suppl 1):S-900.
4. Neto MG, Silva LB, Grecco E, de Quadros LG, Teixeira A, Souza T, Scarparo J, Parada AA, Dib R, Moon R, Campos J. Brazilian Intragastric Balloon Consensus Statement (BIBC): practical guidelines based on experience of over 40,000 cases. Surg Obes Relat Dis. 2018;14(2):151–9.
5. Fittipaldi-Fernandez RJ, Sander B, Galvao Neto MP, Scarparo J, Barrichello S, Diestel CF. Intragastric balloon as a treatment method for excess weight: a large Brazilian experience. Gastroenterology. 2015;148(4, Suppl 1):S-901.

Air-Filled Intragastric Balloon Implant

18

Marcelo Falcão and Maria Cristina Martins

Introduction

The Heliosphere® intragastric balloon (IGB) (Helioscopie Medical Implants, France) is radiopaque, made of a polymer coated with silicone, enclosed in a protective cover, and weighs approximately 30 g (Fig. 18.1). It has a double air pocket that makes monitoring by imaging tests safer. It was licensed for use in Canada in December 2004, but has not been approved in the USA yet [1].

Studies show that the air-filled balloon is efficient and well tolerated and carries a weight loss similar to other types of balloons [2]. In a 12-month follow-up, 30% of patients maintained a weight loss greater than 10% [3]. Regular multidisciplinary follow-up appointments, particularly those related to nutritional and psychological aspects, are central to attain satisfactory long-term results [4, 5].

Indications and Contraindications

The criteria to indicate the intragastric balloon placement are independent of the substance used to fill the device.

M. Falcão (✉)
Surgical Clinic, Baiana School of the Medicine and Health Public, Salvador, BA, Brazil

M. C. Martins
Gastrointestinal Departament, São Rafael Hospital-, Avenida Sáo Rafael, Salvador, BA, Brazil

© Springer Nature Switzerland AG 2020
M. Galvao Neto et al. (eds.), *Intragastric Balloon for Weight Management*,
https://doi.org/10.1007/978-3-030-27897-7_18

Fig. 18.1 Air-filled balloon – Heliosphere BAG®

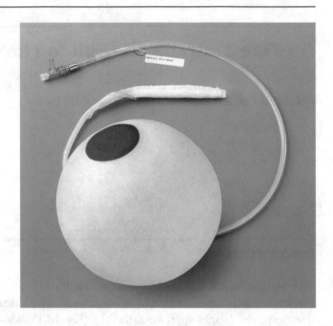

Air-Filled Balloon Placement

The placement and removal of the IGB are endoscopic interventional procedures that should be carried out by a qualified endoscopist familiar with the patient. Preparation for the procedure should be addressed in the first consultation, with a detailed preoperative, multidisciplinary evaluation. Prior to the placement of the IGB, the patient should undergo appropriate preparation, through multidisciplinary evaluation, preoperative exams, informed consent, and routine endoscopy preparation.

Technique

- Monitored anesthesia care preferentially carried out by an anesthesiologist.
- Introduction of the catheter delivery system to the stomach through the mouth.
- The positioning of the balloon below the lower esophageal sphincter should be certified with direct endoscopic visualization (Fig. 18.2).
- The air-filled balloon, after adequate positioning, has a safety system with a polypropylene thread that should be cut to release the protective layer before inflation (Fig. 18.3).
- After removing the thread, the entire white nylon thread is drawn, which opens the protective layer of the balloon.
- The balloon is then filled with 650 to 750 mL of air and released to float freely in the stomach (Fig. 18.4).

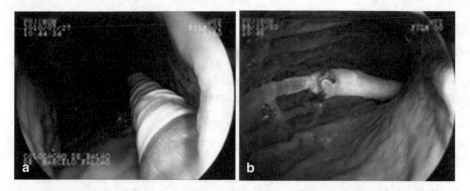

Fig. 18.2 (**a**) Introduction of the IGB in the gastric chamber; (**b**) Positioning of the balloon in the gastric chamber

Fig. 18.3 Connecting tube with safety lock and polypropylene thread

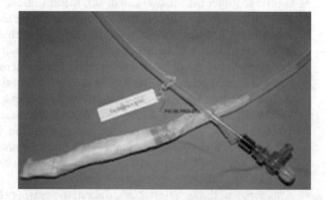

Fig. 18.4 Endoscopic view of balloon filled with air

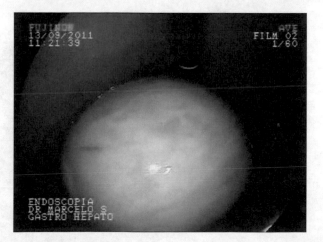

Air-Filled Balloon Removal

As aforementioned, a qualified endoscopist should always be the responsible for the procedure. Planning for removal begins 6 months after the IGB placement with another pre-procedural consultation, as well as multidisciplinary guidance, in order to maintain the lifestyle changes in eating and daily habits.

Technique

- Confirmation of the appropriate removal material supplied by manufacturer.
- Preferably general anesthesia with systematic orotracheal intubation carried out by an anesthesiologist.
- Peroral endoscopy, with the aspiration of possible undigested food in the stomach.
- Gastric chamber insufflation and device identification.
- Multiple punctures in the balloon with a needle catheter.
- Puncture the balloon at the edge of the valve and aspirate all air content.
- Withdrawal of the needle catheter.
- Apprehension of the deflated device with a grasper forceps.
- Positioning and seizing of the IGB at the junction of the valve with the balloon surface for better traction with clamp covering its hook.
- Venous infusion of scopolamine carried out by the anesthesiologist.
- Traction of the balloon toward the esophagogastric junction, avoiding hasty maneuvers or attempting to remove in a single movement.
- The traction must be done in a continuous progressive fashion with rotations of up to 180° of the endoscope-grasper-balloon set.
- After removal through the mouth, discard the grasper (Fig. 18.5).
- Endoscopically check for possible trauma related to the procedure.

Fig. 18.5 Empty balloon and endoscopic tools for removal

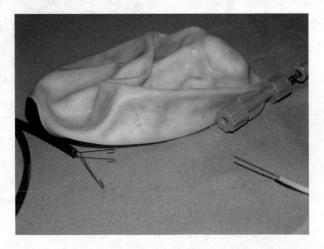

At the end of the endoscopic procedure, the patient remains under monitorization until complete recovery and is then sent to post-anesthetic recovery bed. The post-removal orientation is then reinforced.

Discussion

The intragastric balloon has been increasingly employed for the treatment of obesity and overweight as clinical treatment frequently does not achieve the desired result. Among the existing balloons, the liquid-filled IGB and air-filled Heliosphere® are the most commonly used ones. The treatment with IGB should be reserved for patients who do not meet the criteria for bariatric surgery or who refuse a permanent intervention [6].

Accordingly, a multi-center Brazilian study evaluated 273 patients with air-filled balloons and found a mean excess weight loss of 42%. Therefore, it is concluded that the procedure and the entire treatment are safe and effective compared to the results obtained with liquid-filled IGB [6]. However, in a double-blind study with 20 morbidly obese patients (BMI >40 kg/m^2), Rigaud et al. defined an air-filled balloon group (500 mL) and one without a balloon; both groups underwent similar endoscopic procedures, and both were kept on low-calorie diets during the same follow-up. The authors concluded that the treatment with IGB should not be indicated for morbidly obese patients, as the patients did not achieve significant weight loss [7].

In an evaluation of 32 patients over 4 years, with an 18-month follow-up, Giuricin et al. concluded that the Heliosphere® air-filled balloon generally reduces preoperative risks for bariatric surgery [8]. Between 2005 and 2011, Caglar et al. achieved an absolute weight loss of 13 kg with air-filled IGB in 32 obese (BMI >35 kg/m^2) patients compared to 19 kg obtained with liquid-filled balloons [9].

In a series of 50 patients treated with air-filled balloons between 2005 and 2007, Sciume et al. reported the removal of the device within 24 hours in two patients (4%) due to acute intolerance. The balloons were withdrawn from two other patients (4%) after 5 months of treatment after radiological images showed deflation. The remaining 46 balloons were removed at the end of 6 months, with a positive evaluation of the efficacy, tolerance, and safety of the placement and withdrawal procedures. Patients had an average weight loss of 16.8 kg and a decrease in BMI of 5.9% [10].

Accordingly, Lecumberri et al. evaluated 84 patients during a follow-up of 182 days and recorded a weight loss of 14.5 kg and a BMI reduction of 5.3%; the mean loss of excess weight was 33.2% in this series. Spontaneous deflation (3%) and early surgical removal (1.2%) were also reported as adverse events. However, during the first week, 7.4% of patients suffered from nausea, vomiting, and dyspeptic symptoms [11]. Good tolerance was also observed by Trande et al., who reported the placement procedure to be easy. Nonetheless, dyspeptic symptoms were described for 3 days after the implantation of the air-filled balloons [12]. Serious complications such as gastric distension, spontaneous emptying with intestinal obstruction, erosions, and gastric ulcers are far less common [13, 14].

The removal procedure has been described as more complex, yet feasible and reproducible. De Castro et al. reported some difficulty at this stage due to the resistance of the gastroesophageal junction [2]. Giardello et al. found similar results as the duration of the removal procedure was significantly longer for the Heliosphere® balloon due to the resistance at the cardia and at the distal portion of the pharynx, which conveyed discomfort to patients [15].

Final Considerations

The intragastric balloon appears to be an efficient device for the treatment of overweight and obesity in patients who have not achieved satisfactory results with clinical treatment or who are not fit for or refuse bariatric surgery.

Adverse events may occur during the implantation and removal of the device; therefore the procedure should be carried out by a qualified endoscopist with appropriate equipment.

References

1. Allison C. Intragastric balloons: a temporary treatment for obesity. Issues Emerg Health Technol. 2006;79:1–4.
2. De Castro ML, Morales MJ, Del Campo V, et al. Efficacy, safety, and tolerance of two types of intragastric balloons placed in obese subjects: a double-blind comparative study. Obes Surg. 2010;20(12):1642–6.
3. Mion F, Gincul R, Roman S, et al. Tolerance and efficacy of an air-filled balloon in non-morbidly obese patients: results of a prospective multicenter study. Obes Surg. 2007;17(6):764–9.
4. Geovanelli A. From overweight to super-obesity: the efficacy of air-failled balloon. In: IFSO, XIV World Congress, O-099, 2009, Paris. Anais eletrônicos. Paris, 2009. Disponível em: http://www.helioscopie.fr/sites/default/files/IFSO_2009_abst.pdf. Acesso em: 07 Jul 2013.
5. Balão Intragástrico e Assistência da Equipe multidisciplinar;Endoscopia em Cirurgia da Obesidade, 2008. Ed. Santos.
6. Falcao M, Galvao Neto MP, Campos JM, et al. Air filled balloon – Brazilian Multicentric Study. Obes Surg. 2009;19:953–1076.
7. Rigaud D, Trostler N, Rozen R, et al. Gastric distension, hunger and energy intake after balloon implantation in severe obesity. Int J Obes Relat Metab Disord. 1995;19(7):489–95.
8. Giuricin M, Nagliati C, Palmisano S, et al. Short- and long-term efficacy of intragastric air-filled balloon (Heliosphere(R) BAG) among obese patients. Obes Surg. 2012;22(11):1686–9.
9. Caglar E, Dobrucali A, Bal K. Gastric balloon to treat obesity: filled with air or fluid? Dig Endosc. 2013;25(5):502–7.
10. Sciume C, Geraci G, Pisello F, et al. Role of intragastric air filled ballon (Heliosphere Bag) in severe obesity. Personal experience. Ann Ital Chir. 2009;80(2):113–7.
11. Lecumberri E, Krekshi W, Matia P, et al. Effectiveness and safety of air-filled balloon Heliosphere BAG(R) in 82 consecutive obese patients. Obes Surg. 2011;21(10):1508–12.
12. Trande P, Mussetto A, Mirante VG, et al. Efficacy, tolerance and safety of new intragastric air-filled balloon (Heliosphere BAG) for obesity: the experience of 17 cases. Obes Surg. 2010;20(9):1227–30.
13. Hegade VS, Sood R, Douds AC. Small bowel obstruction induced by spontaneous partial deflation of an intragastric balloon. Ann R Coll Surg Engl. 2012;94(4):e171–3.
14. Moszkowicz D, Lefevre JH. Deflated intragastric balloon-induced small bowel obstruction. Clin Res Hepatol Gastroenterol. 2012;36(1):e17–9.
15. Giardiello C, Borrelli A, Silvestri E, et al. Air-filled vs water-filled intragastric balloon: a prospective randomized study. Obes Surg. 2012;22(12):1916–9.

Part IV

Acute Complications and Treatment

Intolerance to the Device – Abdominal Pain, Nausea, and Others

19

Joseph Sujka, Andre F. Teixeira, Rena Moon, and Muhammad Jawad

Introduction

Postoperative nausea and vomiting are estimated to occur among 25–30% of patients who undergo surgery [1]. These symptoms are mostly secondary to patient exposure to anesthetics or opioid analgesia. The rate of nausea and vomiting in those undergoing intragastric balloon (IGB) placement can be as high as 90% [2]. IGB placement is typically performed in an outpatient setting; however, if severe nausea and vomiting develop, inpatient observation and fluid resuscitation may be necessary. In the case of IGB, nausea and vomiting may continue beyond the postoperative period but typically resolve after 48 hours [2]. If these symptoms fail to improve or resolve after 48 hours, they may represent a patient intolerance to the balloon.

Clinical Presentation

Symptoms consistent with device intolerance include abdominal pain (particularly in the epigastrium and left upper quadrant), nausea, and vomiting, which can lead to dehydration, hypokalemia, and functional renal insufficiency [3]. Pain and reflux may represent gastric ulceration or esophagitis. Patients should be tested for Helicobacter pylori prior to balloon placement and started on a proton pump inhibitor (PPI) after placement of the balloon to help prevent these complications. It has also been suggested that nonsteroidal anti-inflammatory drugs (NSAIDs) should be avoided while the balloon is in place, to prevent life-threatening bleeding [4]. Prolonged symptoms over multiple months can lead to gastroesophageal reflux, esophagitis, and gastric ulceration [5]. Outside the United States, pain

J. Sujka · A. F. Teixeira (✉) · R. Moon · M. Jawad
Department of Bariatric Surgery, Orlando Health Institute, Orlando, FL, USA
e-mail: andre.teixeira@orlandohealth.com

© Springer Nature Switzerland AG 2020
M. Galvao Neto et al. (eds.), *Intragastric Balloon for Weight Management*,
https://doi.org/10.1007/978-3-030-27897-7_19

(34%) is the most common side effect with nausea (29%) and reflux (18%) being common [6]. Studies have suggested that balloon intolerance requiring removal may happen in as little as 3.3% of patients or as many as 20% [7–9]. Asian patients may suffer more greatly from these postoperative side effects and balloon intolerance [7].

Symptoms and Balloon Types

Depending on the type of balloon utilized, the rate of postoperative symptoms and intolerance requiring removal may differ. In a study comparing nonadjustable and adjustable intragastric balloons, patients who received an adjustable balloon had 1 day less of vomiting, though this was not statistically significant. Despite the type of balloon, symptoms of nausea, vomiting, and epigastric pain lasted from 1 to 3 days even with optimal management. As part of the study, patients with a nonadjustable balloon required removal and replacement of their balloon at 6 months to match the adjustable balloon group. After placement of this second balloon, these patients had an additional day of symptoms with resolution at 1 to 4 days [10]. Therefore, in patients receiving a second intragastric balloon, it is prudent to set the expectation that symptoms may be worse and not better than at initial placement.

When comparing saline- and air-filled balloons, one study found that both groups were similar with 50% of patients having epigastric pain, 90% nausea, and 72% having episodes of emesis. These symptoms resolved in most patients 48 hours postoperatively [2]. Another study found that saline-filled balloons, specifically Orbera® (Apollo Endosurgery, Inc., Austin, TX, USA), showed an incidence of pain of 33.7% and nausea of 29% [6]. These rates are very similar to the ReShape® Duo (ReShape Medical Inc., San Clemente, CA, USA), another saline-filled balloon tested in the REDUCE trial [11]. Other studies comparing two types of air-filled balloons found that intolerance requiring removal occurred in 20% of patients and intermittent nausea beyond 3 days was found in 13% of patients [12, 13]. From these trials, it appears that neither air- nor fluid-filled balloons are superior in their rate of postoperative and long-term nausea and vomiting.

Treatment and Prevention

Strategies for mitigating postoperative symptoms can be utilized throughout the placement process, though no specific protocol has been created and validated. Strategies include traditional medications such as proton pump inhibitors, antispasmodic drugs including anticholinergics, and antiemetics, which may be prescribed prophylactically to prevent or minimize nausea and vomiting [6]. The only study specific to IGB placement examined the efficacy of ondansetron or ondansetron combined with midazolam in controlling postoperative nausea. The study showed a 31% decrease in nausea and vomiting symptoms in patients who received both ondansetron and midazolam [14]. The study utilized an ondansetron dose of 8 mg and midazolam dose of 0.075 ug/kg, based on ideal body weight.

If symptoms continue after the fourth postoperative day, patients may require removal of their balloon. This depends on the patient as well as the experience of the operating physician. Conservative management, as mentioned above, may be tried for several weeks if agreed upon by the patient and physician. There is no specific time frame in which a balloon must be removed for intolerance, but the more prolonged the symptoms, the more likely a chronic complication such as gastroesophageal reflux, esophagitis, and gastric ulceration may occur.

Other Device-Related Complications

While nausea and vomiting are the most common symptoms after placement of an intragastric balloon, other uncommon complications may occur. These include pancreatitis and gastric outlet obstruction. There are several case reports that describe acute pancreatitis after intragastric balloon placement and a single case series. One report was of a patient who presented to the hospital on postoperative day three with nausea and vomiting. In addition to these complaints, the patient also stated to have developed pain in the epigastrium that radiated to the back. On CT scan, the patient was found to have compression of the midbody of the pancreas from the balloon resulting in acute pancreatitis [15].

Pancreatitis

Acute pancreatitis may present in the perioperative setting but can also occur at other times. There are reports of presentation from 1 month [16] to 1 year [17] postoperatively. A recent case series examined four patients with acute pancreatitis after IGB placement. Patients were found to have a mean age of 27 ± 2.9 years and presentation at a mean of 2.25 ± 1.25 months postoperatively. CT scan was utilized for diagnosis, which visualized compression of the pancreatic body. The average volume of the intragastric balloon was 607.5 ± 64.5 mL [18]. There is some suggestion that liquid-filled balloons may have a higher rate of pancreatitis with the FDA issuing a letter to health-care providers in 2017 recommending close monitoring of patients who undergo this procedure for pancreatitis.

In patients presenting with nausea, vomiting, and abdominal pain radiating to the back, acute pancreatitis must be in the differential. Laboratory exams such as amylase and lipase, in addition to CT scan, should be performed to make the diagnosis. In the setting of acute pancreatitis related to IGB, prompt removal is warranted. This is most often successful with upper endoscopy.

Gastric Outlet Obstruction

Gastric outlet obstruction is uncommon, with a reported rate of 0.76% [5]. Pancreatitis can occur in combination with gastric outlet obstruction [19]. In comparison to pancreatitis, patients with gastric outlet obstruction tend to present with more acute symptoms. In addition, these patients are unable to tolerate either solid or liquid food. There is no consensus on when this complication tends to present, but case reports exist describing gastric outlet obstruction postoperatively at 2 weeks [20] and 2 months [21].

Once the diagnosis of gastric outlet obstruction is made, removal of the IGB must be considered. Due to the obstruction, and often impaction, the removal procedure can be difficult. In one report, multiple esophagogastroduodenoscopy (EGD) attempts were successful in balloon removal but in another, the patient required laparotomy and gastrotomy for removal [19, 21]. Choice for removal method should be guided by the patient's level of symptoms and hemodynamic stability. A recent meta-analysis of the Orbera® intragastric balloon suggested that the rate of balloon migration was related to the balloon-filling volume (BFV). Patients with a BFV greater than 600 mL had a 0.5% rate of migration versus those with less than 600 mL who had a migration rate of 2.26% [22].

Conclusions

Symptoms related to IGB placement usually occur in most patients, resolving in the first few days. Before the implant procedure, the patient must be informed of this possibility. In cases of severe and lasting symptoms, balloon removal may be considered.

Other complications must be considered when a patient that has an IGB presents with abdominal pain. Acute pancreatitis and gastric outlet obstruction should be ruled out, through laboratory and imaging exams, preventing further complications.

References

1. Watcha MF, White PF. Postoperative nausea and vomiting. Its etiology, treatment, and prevention. Anesthesiology. 1992;77(1):162–84.
2. Giardiello C, Borrelli A, Silvestri E, Antognozzi V, Iodice G, Lorenzo M. Air-filled vs water-filled intragastric balloon: a prospective randomized study. Obes Surg. 2012;22(12):1916–9.
3. Roman S, Napoléon B, Mion F, Bory R-M, Guyot P, D'Orazio H, et al. Intragastric balloon for "non-morbid" obesity: a retrospective evaluation of tolerance and efficacy. Obes Surg. 2004;14(4):539–44.
4. Mojkowska A, Gazdzinski S, Fraczek M, Wyleżoł M. Gastric ulcer hemorrhage – a potential life-threatening complication of intragastric balloon treatment of obesity. Obes Facts. 2017;10(2):153–9.
5. Genco A, Bruni T, Doldi SB, Forestieri P, Marino M, Busetto L, et al. BioEnterics intragastric balloon: the Italian experience with 2,515 patients. Obes Surg. 2005;15(8):1161–4.

6. Abu Dayyeh BK, Edmundowicz SA, Jonnalagadda S, Kumar N, Larsen M, Sullivan S, et al. Endoscopic bariatric therapies. Gastrointest Endosc. 2015;81(5):1073–86.

7. Ganesh R, Rao AD, Baladas HG, Leese T. The bioenteric Intragastric balloon (BIB) as a treatment for obesity: poor results in Asian patients. Singap Med J. 2007;48(3):227–31.

8. Loffredo A, Cappuccio M, De Luca M, de Werra C, Galloro G, Naddeo M, et al. Three years experience with the new intragastric balloon, and a preoperative test for success with restrictive surgery. Obes Surg. 2001;11(3):330–3.

9. Imaz I, Martínez-Cervell C, García-Alvarez EE, Sendra-Gutiérrez JM, González-Enríquez J. Safety and effectiveness of the intragastric balloon for obesity. A meta-analysis. Obes Surg. 2008;18(7):841–6.

10. Genco A, Dellepiane D, Baglio G, Cappelletti F, Frangella F, Maselli R, et al. Adjustable intragastric balloon vs non-adjustable intragastric balloon: case-control study on complications, tolerance, and efficacy. Obes Surg. 2013;23(7):953–8.

11. Ponce J, Woodman G, Swain J, Wilson E, English W, Ikramuddin S, et al. The REDUCE pivotal trial: a prospective, randomized controlled pivotal trial of a dual intragastric balloon for the treatment of obesity. Surg Obes Relat Dis Off J Am Soc Bariatr Surg. 2015;11(4):874–81.

12. De Castro ML, Morales MJ, Del Campo V, Pineda JR, Pena E, Sierra JM, et al. Efficacy, safety, and tolerance of two types of intragastric balloons placed in obese subjects: a double-blind comparative study. Obes Surg. 2010;20(12):1642–6.

13. Mion F, Gincul R, Roman S, Beorchia S, Hedelius F, Claudel N, et al. Tolerance and efficacy of an air-filled balloon in non-morbidly obese patients: results of a prospective multicenter study. Obes Surg. 2007;17(6):764–9.

14. Abdelhamid SA, Kamel MS. A prospective controlled study to assess the antiemetic effect of midazolam following intragastric balloon insertion. J Anaesthesiol Clin Pharmacol. 2014;30(3):383–6.

15. Issa I, Taha A, Azar C. Acute pancreatitis caused by intragastric balloon: a case report. Obes Res Clin Pract. 2016;10(3):340–3.

16. Said F, Robert S, Mansour EK. Pancreatitis and intragastric balloon insertion. Surg Obes Relat Dis Off J Am Soc Bariatr Surg. 2016;12(3):e33–4.

17. Vongsuvanh R, Pleass H, van der Poorten D. Acute necrotizing pancreatitis, gastric ischemia, and portal venous gas complicating intragastric balloon placement. Endoscopy. 2012;44 Suppl 2 UCTN:E383–384.

18. Aljiffry M, Habib R, Kotbi E, Ageel A, Hassanain M, Dahlan Y. Acute pancreatitis: a complication of intragastric balloon. Surg Laparosc Endosc Percutan Tech. 2017;27(6):456–9.

19. Öztürk A, Yavuz Y, Atalay T. A case of duodenal obstruction and pancreatitis due to intragastric balloon. Balkan Med J. 2015;32(3):323–6.

20. Redondo-Cerezo E, Martos-Ruiz V, Matas-Cobos A, Ojeda-Hinojosa M, Martínez-Cara JG, Sánchez-Capilla AD, et al. Gastric outlet obstruction after the insertion of a fully filled intragastric balloon. Rev Esp Enfermedades Dig Organo Of La Soc Esp Patol Dig. 2013;105(2):116–7.

21. Khalaf NI, Rawat A, Buehler G. Intragastric balloon in the emergency department: an unusual cause of gastric outlet obstruction. J Emerg Med. 2014;46(4):e113–6.

22. Kumar N, Bazerbachi F, Rustagi T, McCarty TR, Thompson CC, Galvao Neto MP, et al. The influence of the orbera intragastric balloon filling volumes on weight loss, tolerability, and adverse events: a systematic review and meta-analysis. Obes Surg. 2017;27(9):2272–8.

Impaction of Intragastric Balloon in the Antrum

20

Eduardo Grecco, Marcius Vinicius de Moraes, and Vitor Ottoboni Brunaldi

Introduction

The intragastric balloon (IGB) is a device used to promote weight loss, usually indicated for patients with a body mass index (BMI) not high enough for bariatric surgery or who refuse a surgical intervention, and as an adjuvant therapy for preoperative weight loss in super-obese individuals [1–3]. Despite its minimally invasive characteristic, it is not free of adverse events [4–6].

Clinical Case

This is the case of a 65-year-old female, with a BMI of 52 kg/m^2, chronic kidney failure, chronic obstructive pulmonary disease (COPD), and systemic arterial hypertension (SAH). She underwent placement of a liquid-filled IGB aiming to lose weight in preparation for a bariatric surgery. Thirty days after the procedure, she was admitted to the emergency room with a clinical complaint of vomiting and dyspnea; she was diagnosed with decompensated congestive heart failure after the physical examination.

A computed tomography of the abdomen showed significant gastric distention and the IGB located in the antrum (Figs. 20.1, 20.2, and 20.3).

E. Grecco (✉)
Department of Digestive Surgery, ABC Faculty of Medicine, Santo André, SP, Brazil

M. V. de Moraes
Department of Surgery, Pontifical Catholic University, Goiânia, GO, Brazil

V. O. Brunaldi
Endoscopy Unit of the Department of Gastroenterology, (Hospital das Clínicas da Faculdade de Medicina da Universidade de São Paulo), University of São Paulo (Universidade de São Paulo), São Paulo, SP, Brazil
e-mail: vitor.brunaldi@usp.br

© Springer Nature Switzerland AG 2020
M. Galvao Neto et al. (eds.), *Intragastric Balloon for Weight Management*,
https://doi.org/10.1007/978-3-030-27897-7_20

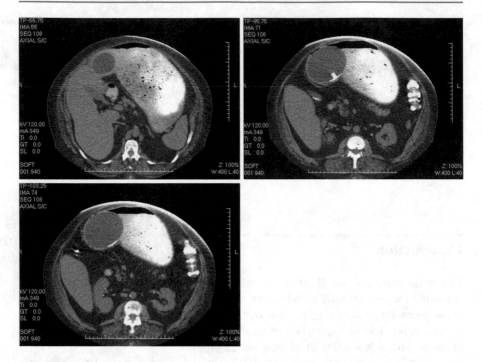

Figs. 20.1, 20.2, and 20.3 Sequence of computer tomography axial sections of the intragastric balloon impacted in the antrum, with gastric distension and accumulation of food residue

Endoscopic Procedure to Remove the Intragastric Balloon

- The procedure was performed in an operating room.
- The patient was positioned in left lateral decubitus, after the anesthesiologist performed general anesthesia and orotracheal intubation.
- A standard single-channel endoscope was introduced, identifying a large amount of solid foods in the gastric body which did not allow visualization of the IGB.
- The endoscope was removed and a Fouchet orogastric tube was used to achieve partial gastric cleaning.
- The endoscope was then reintroduced and advanced to the antrum where the balloon was located (Figs. 20.4 and 20.5).
- The balloon was completely deflated after its puncture with a needle catheter.
- Finally, the balloon was removed using an endoscopic grasper, without complications.

Follow-Up

The patient was sent to an intensive care unit (ICU) for 48 hours and presented adequate clinical recovery (Table 20.1).

Table 20.1 shows the timeline of events

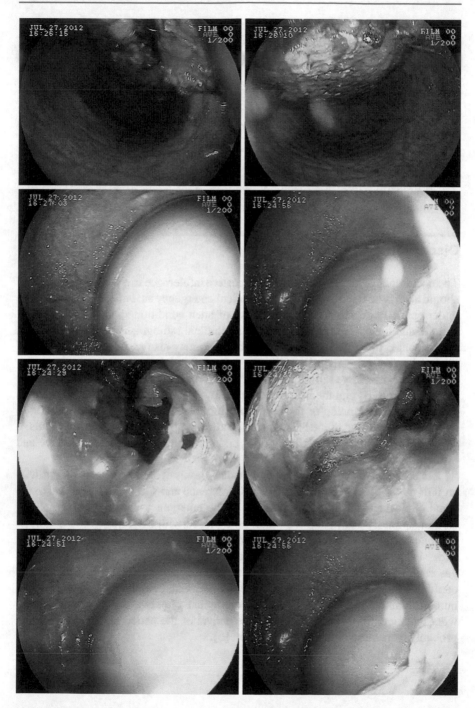

Figs. 20.4 and 20.5 Endoscopic view of the impacted intragastric balloon with a large amount of food residue in the gastric chamber

Table 20.1 Patient's follow-up

	Clinical presentation	Treatment
Day 0	Body mass index = 52 kg/m² Chronic kidney failure Chronic obstructive pulmonary disease Systemic arterial hypertension	Intragastric balloon
30 days	Vomiting and dyspnea Computed tomography of the abdomen Gastric distention IGB impaction in the antrum Upper endoscopy IGB impaction in the antrum	Upper endoscopy Gastric cleaning with a Fouchet catheter Removal of the IGB
30–32 days	Adequate clinical recovery	Observation in the ICU
35 days	Asymptomatic	Hospital discharge

Discussion

The occurrence of abdominal pain and digestive intolerance in a patient with an IGB should always be treated as a potential clinical emergency as it may indicate a severe underlying complication [7]. The workup of such condition should entail at least simple radiological exams such as plain abdominal radiography. In selected cases, the computed tomography (CT) of the abdomen may also assist the assessment of IGB and potential complications.

Vomiting, excessive salivation, and epigastric pain are the most frequent adverse events of the IGB; oral medications are usually enough to control these symptoms and prevent deterioration of the condition. Intractable vomiting may be related to the insufficient filling of the balloon, which allows migration to the antrum. Thus, it significantly impairs the gastric motility and emptying, leading to intolerance and ultimately, early removal [8].

In a case report published in 2012, Ubeda-Iglesias et al. described a patient with an IGB who suffered vomiting and food intolerance and who did not respond to the usual clinical treatment. She was taken to the emergency department, presenting cardiorespiratory arrest, and was finally diagnosed with a severe hydroelectrolytic disorder. After resuscitation and stabilization, a CT of the abdomen revealed an excessive distention of the gastric chamber and the presence of a great amount of gas due to the IGB impaction in the antrum. An upper gastrointestinal endoscopy could identify the balloon and removed it without complications but revealed numerous antral erosions. Although the methylene blue is a good warning sign, it went unnoticed in this case, delaying the arrival of the patient in the hospital and probably worsening of the acute condition [6].

Final Considerations

- Impaction of the IGB in the antrum should always be considered in cases of intractable vomiting, especially in super-obese patients.
- Treatment should be timely, with intravenous hydration, correction of possible hydroelectrolytic disorders, and removal of the IGB when necessary.
- The removal procedure should be performed with caution, because of the risk of bronchial aspiration of the gastric contents.

References

1. Busetto L, Segato G, De Luca M, et al. Preoperative weight loss by intragastric balloon in super-obese patients treated with laparoscopic gastric banding: a case-control study. Obes Surg. 2004;14(5):671–6.
2. Spyropoulos C, Katsakoulis E, Mead N, et al. Intragastric balloon for high-risk super-obese patients: a prospective analysis of efficacy. Surg Obes Relat Dis. 2007;3(1):78–83.
3. Weiner R, Gutberlet H, Bockhorn H. Preparation of extremely obese patients for laparoscopic gastric banding by gastric-balloon therapy. Obes Surg. 1999;9(3):261–4.
4. Al-Zubaidi AM, Alghamdi HU, Alzobydi AH, et al. Bowel perforation due to break and distal passage of the safety ring of an adjustable intra-gastric balloon: a potentially life threatening situation. World J Gastrointest Endosc. 2015;7(4):429–32.
5. Drozdowski R, Wylezol M, Fraczek M, et al. Small bowel necrosis as a consequence of spontaneous deflation and migration of an air-filled intragastric balloon – a potentially life-threatening complication. Wideochir Inne Tech Maloinwazyjne. 2014;9(2):292–6.
6. Ubeda-Iglesias A, Irles-Rocamora JA, Povis-Lopez CD. Antral impaction and cardiorespiratory arrest. Complications of the intragastric balloon. Med Intensiva. 2012;36(4):315–7.
7. Yorke E, Switzer NJ, Reso A, et al. Intragastric balloon for management of severe obesity: a systematic review. Obes Surg. 2016;26(9):2248–54.
8. Papavramidis TS, Grosomanidis V, Papakostas P, et al. Intragastric balloon fundal or antral position affects weight loss and tolerability. Obes Surg. 2012;22(6):904–9.

Intestinal Migration of an Air-Filled Balloon: Laparoscopic Removal

Marcelo Falcão and Flávio Heuta Ivano

Introduction

The intragastric balloon has been used in selected groups of patients who, for one reason or another, are not able to undergo surgical treatment for obesity. However, in spite of its renown as a safe procedure, it is not entirely free from complications. One of the most feared is migration of the balloon.

Among the most common causes of that complication is patient's failure to comply with the 6-month treatment period stipulated by the manufacturer and the medical team. In this chapter, we report a case of intestinal migration of an air-filled balloon treated via laparoscopy.

Clinical Case

A 34-year-old male, BMI 34.6 kg/m^2, with sleep apnea, hepatic steatosis, dyslipidemia, and hypertension was submitted to the implantation of a Heliosphere® (Helioscopie Medical Implants, France) air-filled intragastric balloon.

The patient remained in regular interdisciplinary treatment for 4 months, lost 16 kg, and achieved a BMI of 28.6 kg/m^2. After that, he abandoned the treatment and follow-up and did not reply to calls to come in at the end of 6 months when it was time for the balloon to be removed.

Nine months after the balloon was implanted, he sought out the team complaining of a cramp-like abdominal pain, nausea, uncontrollable vomiting, and feeling bloated. He was referred to the emergency services for examinations.

M. Falcão (✉)
Surgical Clinic, Baiana School of the Medicine and Health Public, Salvador, BA, Brazil

F. H. Ivano
Department of Surgery, Paraná Pontifical Catholic University (PUCPR), Curitiba, PR, Brazil

© Springer Nature Switzerland AG 2020
M. Galvao Neto et al. (eds.), *Intragastric Balloon for Weight Management*,
https://doi.org/10.1007/978-3-030-27897-7_21

An abdominal X-ray revealed distension of intestinal loops in the upper abdomen and balloon impaction in the left iliac fossa (Fig. 21.1). The patient was diagnosed with acute abdomen due to intestinal obstruction from migration of the balloon requiring urgent surgical treatment.

Laparoscopic removal of the intragastric balloon was the choice of management. The inventory of the abdominal cavity showed the distended proximal loop, and the segment with the impaction of the intragastric balloon was identified. The intestine proximal to the balloon was clamped, followed by transverse enterotomy and removal of the balloon under steady aspiration (Fig. 21.2). When part of the intragastric balloon appeared through the abdominal wall, the 12 mm incision was expanded and the balloon cut open with scissors to completely collapse it and, with some slight resistance, it was removed (Fig. 21.3). Enteric contents were aspirated through the enterotomy followed by a longitudinal enterorrhaphy in two layers using absorbable polydioxanone suture thread. Patient was discharged after 3 days based on postoperative ileus status and remained asymptomatic after 2 months with BMI 29.6 kg/m^2.

Fig. 21.1 X-ray image of the abdomen showing the swollen loops of the small intestine in the upper part and the impaction of the balloon in the left iliac quadrant

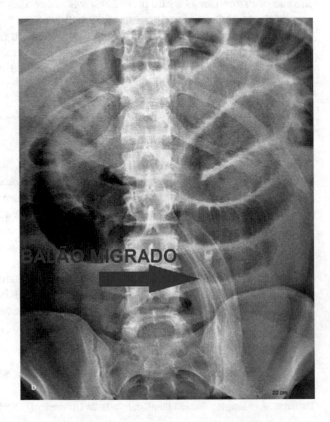

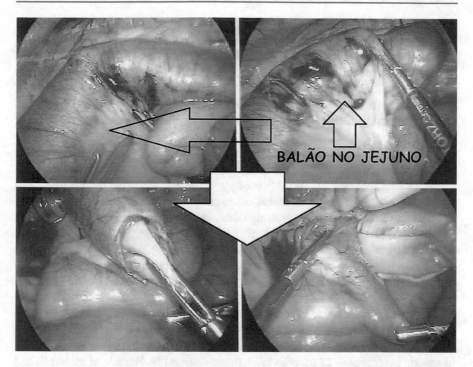

Fig. 21.2 Laparoscopic images of the transverse enterotomy and removal of the intragastric balloon

Fig. 21.3 Laparoscopic image of part of the balloon through the abdominal wall and its complete removal with slight resistance

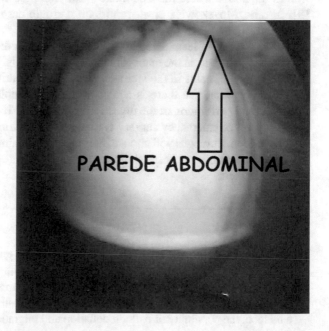

Discussion

The intragastric balloon was designed for temporary use, usually for 6 months, and should it remain implanted for longer than that, it may lead to complications with varying degrees of intensity. Those complications led to the abandonment of the earliest generations of balloon models (Garren–Edwards gastric bubble) and that in turn led to the evolution and definition of the characteristics of an ideal balloon [1, 2].

Those complications were associated to the spontaneous collapse of the balloon and its subsequent migration to the intestine, causing episodes of obstruction. Other complications included the formation of peptic ulcers, digestive hemorrhage, and acute pancreatitis [2–4]. More recent development of the device has considerably reduced those risks but has not entirely eliminated them [4, 5].

The clinical centers that commonly make use of intragastric balloons have reported that migration of the balloon is one of the possible complications and that was particularly true of the early models. Most of the reports concern patients who remained with the balloon implanted beyond the period stipulated by the manufacturer [4].

Zdichavsky et al. describe the migration of a balloon 1 year after implantation when the patient presented an acute abdomen condition associated to intestinal obstruction [6]. There is also a description of a balloon migration associated to gastric perforation, 22 months after implantation [7]. Hegade et al. published a case of migration involving an air-filled balloon with a similar clinical condition to the above where the treatment option adopted was laparoscopic surgery [8]. In turn, Moszkowicz et al. report on a single case involving laparoscopic treatment [9].

The interaction of team members and follow-up after the implantation procedure are an obligatory part in the management of such patients. The period that the intragastric balloon remains in the stomach must not exceed that recommended by the manufacturer otherwise there is a risk of serious complications such as balloon migration and perforation of the digestive system [4, 7, 10].

The object of emergency surgery is to solve the obstruction problem by removing the balloon. Surgeons will choose their method of gaining access to the abdominal cavity according to their skills and qualifications and the structure that is available to them.

Conclusions

- The intragastric balloon is an efficacious device that guarantees good results but to achieve them, the patient must adhere to the manufacturer and medical team's recommendations, thereby avoiding any eventual complications.
- Given a patient condition compatible with intestinal obstruction and the presence of a balloon, the possibility of balloon deflation and migration must be considered.

References

1. Schapiro M, Benjamin S, Blackburn G, et al. Obesity and the gastric balloon: a comprehensive workshop. Tarpon Springs, Florida, March 19–21, 1987. Gastrointest Endosc. 1987;33(4):323–7.
2. Nieben OG, Harboe H. Intragastric balloon as an artificial bezoar for treatment of obesity. Lancet. 1982;1(8265):198–9.
3. Sallet JA, Marchesini JB, Paiva DS, et al. Brazilian multicenter study of the intragastric balloon. Obes Surg. 2004;14(7):991–8.
4. Galvão Neto M, Santana MF, Marchesini JCD, et al. Balão intragástrico e assistência da equipe multidisciplinar. In: Campos JM, Galvão Neto MP, EGH M, editors. (Org.). Endoscopia em Cirurgia da Obesidade. Endoscopia em Cirurgia da Obesidade, vol. vol 1. 1st ed. São Paulo: Santos; 2008. p. 1.
5. Evans JD, Scott MH. Intragastric balloon in the treatment of patients with morbid obesity. Br J Surg. 2001;88(9):1245–8.
6. Zdichavsky M, Beckert S, Kueper M, et al. Mechanical ileus induces surgical intervention due to gastric balloon: a case report and review of the literature. Obes Surg. 2010;20(12):1743–6.
7. Baigel R, Rashid F, Shrestha D, et al. Peritonitis following a bariatric procedure in a young woman. BMJ Case Rep. 2011;2011:bcr1220103602.
8. Hegade VS, Sood R, Douds AC. Small bowel obstruction induced by spontaneous partial deflation of an intragastric balloon. Ann R Coll Surg Engl. 2012;94(4):e171–3.
9. Moszkowicz D, Lefevre JH. Deflated intragastric balloon-induced small bowel obstruction. Clin Res Hepatol Gastroenterol. 2012;36(1):e17–9.
10. Smigielski JA, Szewczyk T, Modzelewski B, et al. Gastric perforation as a complication after BioEnterics intragastric balloon bariatric treatment in obese patients–synergy of endoscopy and videosurgery. Obes Surg. 2010;20(11):1597–9.

Migration of the Liquid-Filled Balloon: Intestinal Sub-occlusion

22

Victor Ramos Mussa Dib, Lyz Bezerra Silva, and Josemberg M. Campos

Introduction

In spite of the technical ease of placement of the intragastric balloon and its tolerance by patients, the risk of complications such as deflation and migration to the small intestine does exist, and it increases the longer the balloon remains in place. Most authors recommend removal of the device after 6 months; most of the migration events reported occur after that period [1].

This chapter reports the case of the spontaneous deflation of an intragastric balloon that occurred 4 months after its implantation and describes the surgical procedure adopted for management.

Clinical Case

A 36-year-old woman, BMI 29 kg/m^2, with no comorbidities was submitted to the implantation of an intragastric balloon (Silimed®, Rio de Janeiro, Brasil), which was then filled with liquid. She progressed satisfactorily during the first 4 months of follow-up. Subsequently, she failed to appear for the scheduled consultations and only reappeared 9 months after implantation. On that occasion, she reported having been in pain for 4 days with cramps, nausea, flatulence, and distension followed by

V. R. M. Dib (✉)
Department of Surgery, Victor Dib Institute, Manaus, AM, Brazil

L. B. Silva · J. M. Campos
Department of Surgery, Federal University of Pernambuco, Recife, PE, Brazil

© Springer Nature Switzerland AG 2020
M. Galvao Neto et al. (eds.), *Intragastric Balloon for Weight Management*,
https://doi.org/10.1007/978-3-030-27897-7_22

bouts of diarrhea. It was not possible to feel the presence of the balloon by physical examination.

An abdominal ultrasound was not able to visualize the balloon, while a tomography showed thickening in the distal ileum and moderate swelling of small intestine. An abdominal X-ray showed the migrated prosthesis present in the ileum (Fig. 22.1).

After this finding, surgical management by laparoscopy was chosen. The balloon was found lodged in the terminal ileum presenting a tubular aspect and causing thickening of the walls of the loop and slight distension (Fig. 22.2). Given the proximity of the cecum, it was not possible to resect the intestinal segment containing the balloon because it would then be necessary to restructure the passage by means of an ileocolonic anastomosis. On the other hand, simply opening the intestinal loop and extracting the prosthesis would lead to a gross contamination of the cavity. The option was for a combined procedure making use of a prior Pfannenstiel incision, pulling the intestinal loop outside of the abdominal cavity. An enterotomy was performed, allowing removal of the balloon (Figs. 22.3 and 22.4).

The patient progressed without any occurrences and was discharged from hospital in 24 hours.

Fig. 22.1 Simple X-ray image of the abdomen showing the deflated migrated balloon lodged in the distal ileum (white arrows)

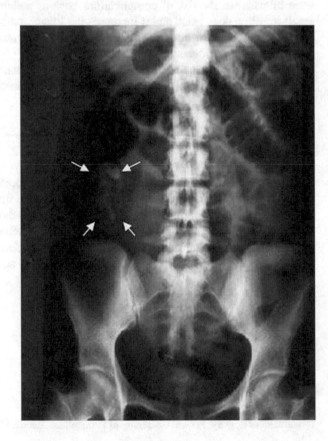

Fig. 22.2 Laparoscopic view of the migrated balloon

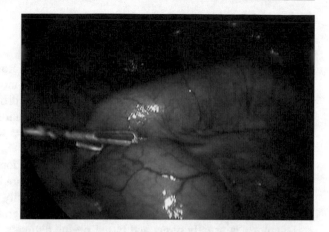

Fig. 22.3 Enterotomy and removal of the balloon

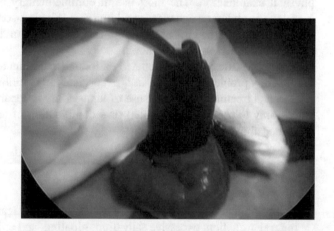

Fig. 22.4 Suturing of the bowel

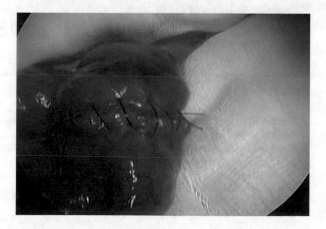

Discussion

Vomiting, regurgitation, excessive salivation, bloating, and epigastralgia are the complications most frequently associated to intragastric balloons, and they generally occur in the first 2 weeks after implantation. Other more serious complications that can also occur are gastric ulcer, severe intolerance, difficulties in the process of placing and removing the device, and spontaneous deflation [1–5]. One of the most serious complications is intestinal obstruction that occurs when the balloon deflates spontaneously and passes into the small intestine [6].

Liquid-filled balloons are filled with a saline solution mixed with methylene blue, which causes the urine to turn green if the liquid should happen to escape from the balloon. It is essential that the patient should be fully informed regarding that possibility, thereby reducing the risk of an intestinal migration [7].

Diagnosis is usually direct and based on the patient's anamnesis and a careful physical examination. The most useful complementary examination is a simple X-ray of the abdomen and ultrasound imaging [8]. Non-contrasted tomography can also help because the air and the liquid in the bowels provide a perfect contrast for the radio-opaqueness of the balloon.

While it is true that some deflated balloons are eliminated via the digestive tract without any problems, in most cases, a surgical intervention is necessary [9].

Surgical treatment can make use of laparotomy or laparoscopy (carrying out an enterotomy to remove the balloon) or a combination of techniques as in the case described above [1, 4].

Final Remarks

- The complications most frequently associated to intragastric balloons are vomiting, regurgitation, excessive salivation, bloating, and epigastralgia.
- One of the most serious complications is intestinal obstruction caused by spontaneous deflation of the balloon.
- Intestinal obstruction caused by a migrated balloon is usually treated with a surgical intervention.

References

1. Vanden Eynden F, Urbain P. Small intestine gastric balloon impaction treated by laparoscopic surgery. Obes Surg. 2001;11(5):646–8.
2. Genco A, Bruni T, Doldi SB, et al. BioEnterics intragastric balloon: the Italian experience with 2,515 patients. Obes Surg. 2005;15(8):1161–4.
3. Koutelidakis I, Dragoumis D, Papaziogas B, et al. Gastric perforation and death after the insertion of an intragastric balloon. Obes Surg. 2009;19(3):393–6.
4. Matar ZS, Mohamed AA, Abukhater M, et al. Small bowel obstruction due to air-filled intragastric balloon. Obes Surg. 2009;19(12):1727–30.

5. Sanchez-Perez MA, Munoz-Juarez M, Cordera-Gonzalez de Cosio F, et al. Gastric perforation and subarachnoid hemorrhage secondary to intragastric balloon device. Rev Gastroenterol Mex. 2011;76(3):264–9.
6. Hegade VS, Sood R, Douds AC. Small bowel obstruction induced by spontaneous partial deflation of an intragastric balloon. Ann R Coll Surg Engl. 2012;94(4):e171–3.
7. Bernante P, Francini F, Zangrandi F, et al. Green urine after intragastric balloon placement for the treatment of morbid obesity. Obes Surg. 2003;13(6):951–3.
8. Francica G, Giardiello C, Iodice G, et al. Ultrasound as the imaging method of choice for monitoring the intragastric balloon in obese patients: normal findings, pitfalls and diagnosis of complications. Obes Surg. 2004;14(6):833–7.
9. Mousavi Naeini SM, Sheikh M. Bowel obstruction due to migration of an intragastric balloon necessitating surgical removal before completion of the recommended 6 months. Case Rep Med. 2012;2012:414095.

Gastric Perforation by Intragastric Balloon

23

Victor Ramos Mussa Dib, Lyz Bezerra Silva, and Josemberg M. Campos

Introduction

The implantation of an intragastric balloon as part of the treatment for obesity is a minimally invasive therapy originally proposed by Nieben and Harboe in the 1980s [1, 2].

In spite of the noninvasive nature of the procedure, complications may sometimes occur, such as intolerance, gastric obstruction, gastric ulcer, and gastric perforations [3]. Their occurrence motivated the holding of a conference in 1987, which established the basic requirements for an intragastric balloon, one of which was that it should have a very smooth surface with little propensity to cause ulceration [4].

Although the balloons used today are very safe, they are not entirely free from the risk of complications [5]. Here, we describe a case of gastric perforation in the presence of an intragastric balloon and its treatment using laparoscopy.

V. R. M. Dib (✉)
Department of Surgery, Victor Dib Institute, Manaus, AM, Brazil

L. B. Silva · J. M. Campos
Department of Surgery, Federal University of Pernambuco, Recife, PE, Brazil

© Springer Nature Switzerland AG 2020
M. Galvao Neto et al. (eds.), *Intragastric Balloon for Weight Management*,
https://doi.org/10.1007/978-3-030-27897-7_23

Clinical Case

A woman, BMI 28.7 kg/m^2, was submitted to the implantation of an intragastric balloon (Silimed®, Rio de Janeiro, Brazil). She progressed satisfactorily during the entire period of monthly medical and multidisciplinary follow-up and lost 14 kg. A proton pump inhibiting drug was prescribed for as long as the balloon was in place, but administration was suspended in the fifth month in accordance with the protocol adopted by the clinic. Toward the end of the treatment period, a little before the planned removal of the balloon, the patient suddenly experienced acute epigastric pain and had to be hospitalized and treated with opioids.

Laboratory exams, thorax, and abdominal X-ray showed no alterations. Also, an abdominal ultrasound was performed, with no abnormal findings.

An endoscopy was then performed, which showed difficulty to stretch the stomach for the deflation maneuver and impossibility of assessing other alterations due to the presence of the balloon, and removal of the intragastric balloon was performed.

At the end of the endoscopic examination, the clinical examination detected an intense abdominal distension consistent with pneumoperitoneum, which was confirmed by an X-ray of the abdomen. A new upper gastrointestinal tract endoscopy was performed and a perforated ulcer on the anterior wall of the stomach was detected.

A laparoscopy was then performed, which showed an oval, straight-edged perforation on the anterior wall of the stomach with a diameter of approximately 15 mm (Fig. 23.1) and a small amount of serofibrinous secretion in the cavity. The lesion was sutured with individual stitches using polypropylene 3.0 thread (Fig. 23.2), and epiplonplasty and rinsing/aspiration of the cavity were done (Fig. 23.3).

The patient progressed satisfactorily and was discharged from the hospital 48 hours later, remaining asymptomatic on follow-up.

Fig. 23.1 Laparoscopic view of the perforation in the anterior gastric wall

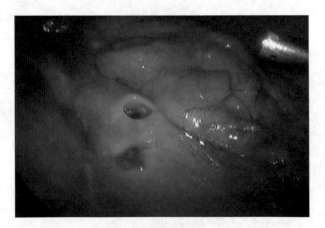

Fig. 23.2 Suture of the
lesion with individual
stitches of 3.0
polypropylene thread

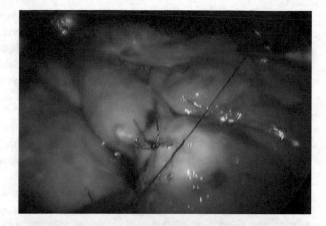

Fig. 23.3 Omental patch

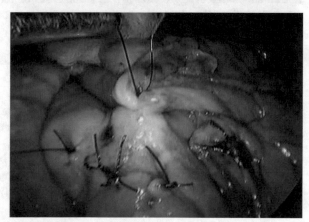

Discussion

The formation of ulcers and gastric erosions in the presence of an intragastric balloon can be associated to irritation of the stomach wall and cytoprotection failure,
secondary to the production of prostaglandins by the mucosa. The presence of food
residues squeezed between the wall and the balloon and/or the irregular surface of
the balloon valve may create a zone of high pressure and ischemia and eventually
culminate with a perforation, albeit that complication is rare [6].

A history of previous gastric surgery with the associated reduction in the organ's
complacency constitutes a definitive contraindication for the placement of an intragastric balloon [3, 7]. In a series of 2515 patients, only 5 presented the complication of perforation. Of those five, four had previously undergone Nissen
fundoplication surgery and in two cases, the patients died. In the said series, the
rate of occurrence of perforation in patients with a history of previous gastric surgery was 66.6% [3].

Sudden acute abdominal pain occurring days or even months after intragastric balloon placement is a sign of a possible gastric perforation, a serious complication that can lead to sepsis and death if it is not diagnosed early on [8, 9]. The diagnosis is based on the clinical findings with a special focus on intense epigastric pain, on the physical examination, abdominal tympanism, and abdominal defense, depending on the stage of the complication at which the diagnosis is being made.

In some cases, the intragastric balloon may block the perforated area thereby preventing the formation of a pneumoperitoneum and delaying prompt diagnosis. The definitive etiological diagnosis is obtained by endoscopy, which is routinely performed after removal of the balloon.

The definitive treatment is a surgical intervention to close the perforation and clean the cavity [10]. Whenever possible, videolaparoscopy is the preferred method, minimizing surgical aggression [8]. In some cases of very small perforations, with no evident clinical repercussions, an endoscopic intervention for the placement of clips and sutures may be a viable option.

Final Remarks

- The possibility of a gastric perforation must be considered in cases where a patient with an intragastric balloon implanted experiences sudden, acute abdominal pain.
- Endoscopy provides the definitive diagnosis but can be complemented by X-ray and ultrasound examinations and by computerized tomography.
- Treatment of this complication is urgent and usually via surgical intervention closing the lesion and cleaning the cavity.

References

1. Nieben OG, Harboe H. Intragastric balloon as an artificial bezoar for treatment of obesity. Lancet. 1982;1(8265):198–9.
2. Harboe H, Nieben OG. Intragastric balloon in the treatment of obesity. Report of a pilot study. Ugeskr Laeger. 1982;144(6):394–6.
3. Genco A, Bruni T, Doldi SB, et al. BioEnterics intragastric balloon: the Italian experience with 2,515 patients. Obes Surg. 2005;15(8):1161–4.
4. Schapiro M, Benjamin S, Blackburn G, et al. Obesity and the gastric balloon: a comprehensive workshop. Tarpon Springs, Florida, March 19–21, 1987. Gastrointest Endosc. 1987;33(4):323–7.
5. Yorke E, Switzer NJ, Reso A, et al. Intragastric balloon for management of severe obesity: a systematic review. Obes Surg. 2016;26(9):2248–54.
6. Koutelidakis I, Dragoumis D, Papaziogas B, et al. Gastric perforation and death after the insertion of an intragastric balloon. Obes Surg. 2009;19(3):393–6.
7. Giardiello C, Cristiano S, Cerbone MR, et al. Gastric perforation in an obese patient with an intragastric balloon, following previous fundoplication. Obes Surg. 2003;13(4):658–60.

8. Abou Hussein BM, Khammas AA, Al Ani AM, et al. Gastric perforation following intragastric balloon insertion: combined endoscopic and laparoscopic approach for management: case series and review of literature. Obes Surg. 2016;26(5):1127–32.
9. Al-Zubaidi AM, Alghamdi HU, Alzobydi AH, et al. Bowel perforation due to break and distal passage of the safety ring of an adjustable intragastric balloon: a potentially life threatening situation. World J Gastrointest Endosc. 2015;7(4):429–32.
10. Sanchez-Perez MA, Munoz-Juarez M, Cordera-Gonzalez de Cosio F, et al. Gastric perforation and subarachnoid hemorrhage secondary to intragastric balloon device. Rev Gastroenterol Mex. 2011;76(3):264–9.

Hyperinflated Intragastric Balloon

24

Thiago Ferreira de Souza, Eduardo Grecco, and Eduardo N. Usuy Jr.

Introduction

Weight reduction in obese patients and the subsequent maintenance of weight loss can significantly improve the quality of life and decrease the impact of associated comorbidities. Lifestyle-based interventions such as healthy eating habits and regular physical activity are often ineffective in ensuring not only weight loss but also long-term maintenance of weight loss [1, 5].

With the increase of obesity in the world, nonsurgical techniques have been developed to reduce body weight, such as the implantation of an intragastric balloon (IGB). The idea came from the observation that psychiatric patients who presented gastric bezoars also experienced weight loss [1]. The first balloons were composed of gum and latex but the patients suffered from sudden rupture and emptying. Therefore, they were posteriorly replaced by polyurethane balloons inflated with air [2] and ultimately by the "bioenterics IGB" (Orbera® Apollo Endosurgery, Inc., Austin, TX, USA) that has similar a structure to the one used currently [3].

The IGB is a sphere made of a silicone elastomer that is filled with between 400 and 700 mL of 0.9% saline solution and methylene blue. The balloon, which is implanted in the stomach through an endoscopic procedure, also has a radiopaque valve that is connected to a catheter for filling [1, 3]. Subsequently, it is positioned in the gastric fundus where it reduces the intragastric volume, suppressing hunger and increasing satiety (Fig. 24.1). The IGB should remain in the stomach for around

T. F. de Souza (✉)
Director of Instituto Endovitta, ABC Medical School, Santo Paulo, SP, Brazil

E. Grecco
Department of Digestive Surgery, ABC Faculty of Medicine, Santo André, SP, Brazil

E. N. Usuy Jr.
Department of Gastroenterology and Bariatric Endoscopy, Gástrica Clínic, Florianópolis, SC, Brazil
e-mail: usuy@usuy.com.br

© Springer Nature Switzerland AG 2020
M. Galvao Neto et al. (eds.), *Intragastric Balloon for Weight Management*,
https://doi.org/10.1007/978-3-030-27897-7_24

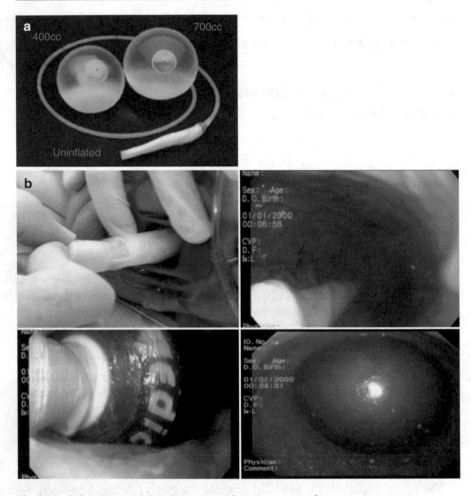

Fig. 24.1 Inflated intragastric balloon (**a**) and insertion process (**b**)

6 months after which time there is an increased risk of complications, such as rupture and migration [1–4]. Several types of IGB are currently available on the market (Table 24.1).

The IGB is implanted endoscopically during a minimally invasive, temporary, and completely reversible procedure. It is a safe modality of treatment with good results reported in the literature for weight loss in the adult population [5–7].

In an Italian study enrolling 2515 patients, Genco et al. reported an overall complication rate of 2.8% (70 patients). Gastric perforation occurred in five patients (0.19%), 19 suffered from gastric obstruction (0.76%), rupture of the balloon occurred in 0.36%, esophagitis in 1.27%, and gastric ulcers in 0.2% (40 patients) [9, 10].

Rarely, fungal colonization of the IGB and its content may be observed. However, the patient remains asymptomatic in most cases [11–13]. During removal, whitish lumps may be observed on the surface of the balloon. It is hypothesized that

Table 24.1 Types of intragastric balloon

	Intragastric liquid balloon	Double balloon system	Adjustable intragastric balloon	Obalon intragastric balloon
Characteristics	Single silicone balloon (450–700 mL) Filled with saline solution and methylene blue [4]	Two connected balloons ("double balloon") (450 mL each) Filled with saline solution and methylene blue [4]	Single adjustable silicone balloon Filled with saline solution alone or with methylene blue [4]	Digestible gelatinous capsule (250 mL) Single balloon inflated with Nitrogen gas [4]
Implantation	Endoscopy	Endoscopy	Endoscopy	Digested and monitored by X-ray
Removal	After 6 months [5]	After 6 months [5]	After 12 months[a]	After 3 months [5]

[a]According to the manufacturer

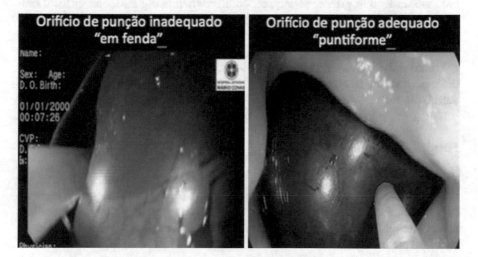

Fig. 24.2 Inadequate and adequate puncture of the intragastric balloon for emptying

contamination may occur during the placement procedure. The use of proton pump inhibitors, the reduction of gastric acidity, and delayed gastric emptying caused by the balloon might favor this condition [11]. In some cases, hyperinflation of the balloon is also noticed. This situation is usually difficult during the extraction of the balloon, since the puncture and adequate emptying may be more demanding (Fig. 24.2).

Candida albicans is the most commonly found pathogen on the siliconized surfaces, as reported by da Silveira et al. [14]. Usually, the patient remains asymptomatic with this condition, which is only diagnosed during endoscopy. However, the patient may experience nausea, difficult-to-treat vomiting, and abdominal distension. After the removal of the balloon, the patient presents a complete resolution of the symptoms [14].

Epidemiology/Causes

The possible causes for gaseous overfilling/hyperinflation of the balloon are outlined below.

Iatrogenic

If the assistant incorrectly fills the device, with either air or liquid, it may be necessary to remove the balloon immediately depending on the amount inflated. The supplier only guarantees the safety of the balloon up to 700 mL in volume. Therefore, the endoscopist should remove or partially empty the balloon (if the adjustable type) in case of inadequate filling.

Some endoscopists intentionally employ a larger volume than recommended by the supplier, which is empirical and off-label. The idea is that the greater volume would lead to greater satiety, especially when using a second or third balloon in a sequence. However, in our experience, there is no significant difference in either final weight loss or in the posttreatment weight maintenance. This is different from the rationale of the adjustable balloon, for which the supplier guarantees the balloon filled up to 1000 mL. This balloon can be refilled during the period of the treatment in order to maintain satiety for longer than the standard balloon.

Fungal Contamination

The contamination of the IGB and its contents raises the hypothesis that fungal contamination produces gas due to a fermentation process resulting in an increase in its diameter. Ultimately, it leads to obstructive symptoms (nausea, vomiting, ulcers, ischemia, and perforations). In these situations, the balloon should be removed but no topical or systemic drug treatment is required [15].

Pathophysiology

The extremely low incidence of colonization is multifactorial: Gastric stasis, smoking, and the use of antacids are risk factors for opportunistic infections. Colonization is more common on the outer surface of the balloon, and it is only found at the time of the IGB removal, as the patient usually remains asymptomatic (Fig. 24.3). Sometimes the physical characteristics of the IGB are affected making it hard and brittle, occasionally hindering its removal. When patients are symptomatic, they are generally nonspecific such as epigastric pain, vomiting, and in more severe cases, dysphagia due to esophageal colonization.

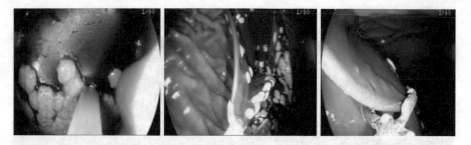

Fig. 24.3 Fungal colonization of the balloon

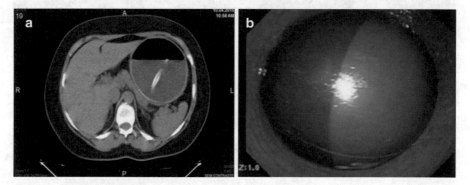

Fig. 24.4 Computed tomography (**a**) and endoscopy (**b**) showing overinflation of the balloon

Case Report

A 37-year-old female patient (height: 1.58 m; weight: 87.5 kg; body mass index: 35 kg/m²) had a history of unsuccessful attempts to lose weight by dieting and medications over 2 years. After an evaluation of a multidisciplinary team, treatment using the 1-year readjustable IGB was indicated.

After the initial period of adaptation, the patient presented a satisfactory weight loss of 12.6 kg (BMI 30 kg/m²). However, by the end of the second month of treatment, she presented with epigastric pain and discomfort after eating, associated with vomiting. Computed tomography revealed abnormal inflation of the balloon (Fig. 24.4). An upper gastrointestinal endoscopy showed an overinflated balloon with a marked fluid-gas level with about 50% of the balloon filled with gas (Fig. 24.4).

We decided to empty the adjustable balloon entirely and sent the first 50 mL for culture (which identified *candida* sp.). Then, we filled up the IGB with 10 mL of nystatin (1,000,000 UI) and 600 mL of methylene blue solution (Fig. 24.5).

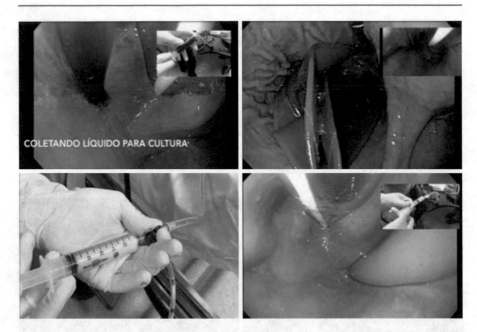

Fig. 24.5 Collecting of the liquid for culture, total emptying of the balloon, and refilling with methylene blue and nystatin solution

Fig. 24.6 Six-month control image of balloon treatment

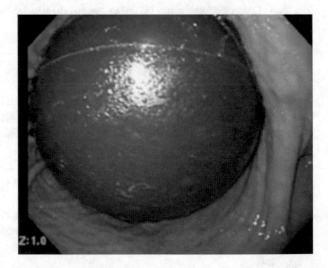

Endoscopic follow-up showed the balloon well placed in the gastric fundus and no gas (Fig. 24.6). She was kept on multidisciplinary counseling with nutrition and endoscopy staff, but no further adjustment was needed. After 6 months, the patient had an asymptomatic weight of 68 kg with a BMI of 27.24; the absolute weight loss was 19.5 kg (% total weight loss = 22.28%). The balloon was removed 12 months after placement without any evidence of further hyperinflation and with the patient asymptomatic.

Treatment

The IGB has a silicone elastomer structure and *in vitro* studies have reported that its silicone-based coating is susceptible to colonization by *candida* [7]. Candidiasis of the gastrointestinal tract mainly affects the esophagus, which presents as white or grayish plaques on the mucosa [8]. Although the typical fungal infection is usually not detected in the esophagus of patients, it cannot be excluded. Contamination of the IGB may occur during endoscopic interventions, that is, during the passage of the device through the oral cavity.

Oral nystatin suspension has an *in vitro* fungicidal action against a wide variety of yeasts and yeast-like fungi. The *Streptomyces noursei* produces this drug. It acts by bonding with steroids in the cell membrane of susceptible fungi, which increases the permeability of the cell membrane and ultimately leads to extravasation of the cytoplasmic content. In repeat subcultures with increasing concentrations of nystatin, the candida albicans does not develop resistance to nystatin. Furthermore, nystatin resistance usually does not appear during treatment, and it has no activity against bacteria, protozoa, or viruses. Nystatin has negligible absorption in the gastrointestinal tract and it is eliminated unchanged in stools.

The option to treat fungal contamination of the IBG with emptying and refilling with nystatin and methylene blue solution is an innovative approach based on the rationale of controlling the infection locally. This approach has been successful without the recurrence of hyperinflation in our practice.

Conclusion

Fungal contamination of the outer surface of the balloon and its liquid content may lead to fermentation and hyperinflation. We propose a randomized clinical trial to evaluate the efficacy of adding nystatin to the balloon solution as prophylaxis against fungal colonization. Preliminary results point to less colonization of the outer surface of the balloon and to a decreased early removal rate.

References

1. Carvalho MR, Jorge Z, Nobre E, et al. Balão intragástrico no tratamento da obesidade mórbida. Acta Med Port. 2011;24:489–98.
2. Swidnicka-Siergiejko A, Wróblewski E, Dabrowski A. Endoscopic treatment of obesity. Can J Gastroenterol. 2011;25(11):627–33.
3. Kethu SR, Banerjee S, Barth BA, et al. Endoluminal bariatric techniques. Gastrointest Endosc. 2012;76(1):1–7.
4. Yap Kannan R, Nutt MR. Are intra-gastric adjustable balloon system safe? A case series. Int J Surg Case Rep. 2013;4(10):936–8.
5. ASGE Bariatric Endoscopy Task Force and ASGE Technology Committee, Abu Dayyeh BK, Kumar N, Edmundowicz SA, Jonnalagadda S, Larsen M, Sullivan S, Thompson CC, Banerjee S. ASGE Bariatric Endoscopy Task Force systematic review and meta-analysis assessing the ASGE PIVI thresholds for adopting endoscopic bariatric therapies. Gastrointest Endosc. 2015;82(3):425–38.e5. https://doi.org/10.1016/j.gie.2015.03.1964. Epub 2015 Jul 29. PubMed PMID: 26232362.

6. Kumar N. Endoscopic therapy for weight loss: gastroplasty, duodenal sleeves, intragastric balloons, and aspiration. World J Gastrointest Endosc. 2015;7(9):847–59. https://doi.org/10.4253/wjge.v7.i9.847. Review. PubMed PMID: 26240686; PubMed Central PMCID: PMC4515419.

7. Zheng Y, Wang M, He S, Ji G. Short-term effects of intragastric balloon in association with conservative therapy on weight loss: a meta-analysis. J Transl Med. 2015;13:246. https://doi.org/10.1186/s12967-015-0607-9. PubMed PMID: 26219459; PubMed Central PMCID: PMC4517653.

8. Angrisani L, Lorenzo M, Borrelli V, Giuffre M, Fonderico C, Capece G. Is bariatric surgery necessary after intragastric balloon treatment? Obes Surg. 2006;16(9):1135–7.

9. Nguyen N, Champion JK, Ponce J, Quebbemann B, Patterson E, Pham B, et al. A review of unmet needs in obesity management. Obes Surg. 2012;22(6):956–66.

10. Genco A, Bruni T, Doldi SB, Forestieri P, Marino M, Busetto L, et al. BioEnterics intragastric balloon: the Italian experience with 2,515 patients. Obes Surg. 2005;15(8):1161–4.

11. Coskun H, Bozkurt S. A case of asymptomatic fungal and bacterial colonization of an intragastric balloon. World J Gastroenterol. 2009;15(45):5751–3.

12. Simsek Z, Gurbuz OA, Coban S. Fungal colonization of intragastric balloons. Endoscopy. 2014;46(Suppl 1 UCTN):E642–3.

13. Kotzampassi K, Vasilaki O, Stefanidou C, Grosomanidis V. Candida albicans colonization on an intragastric balloon. Asian J Endosc Surg. 2013;6(3):214–6.

14. da Silveira LC, Charone S, Maia LC, Soares RM, Portela MB. Biofilm formation by Candida species on silicone surfaces and latex pacifier nipples: an in vitro study. J Clin Pediatr Dent. 2009;33(3):235–40.

15. Kliemann DA, Pasqualotto AC, Falavigna M, Giaretta T, Severo LC. Candida esophagitis: species distribution and risk factors for infection. Rev Inst Med Trop Sao Paulo. 2008;50(5):261–3.

Problems in the Implantation of the Intragastric Balloon

Sérgio Alexandre Barrichello Júnior
and Luiz Gustavo de Quadros

Introduction

Widely used in Brazil for many years, the intragastric balloon (IGB) is an excellent nonsurgical alternative for weight loss [1]. Some measures are necessary to guarantee the safety of the placement procedure. It must be performed in a controlled environment with the adequate equipment and in good conditions. Some specific endoscopic accessories such as foreign body removal forceps, needle, polypectomy snare (large diameter), endoscopic scissors, and overtube are essential to solve possible difficulties. Dabrowiecki et al. described no complications during IGB placement in morbidly obese patients in preparation for bariatric surgery when the procedure was performed under general anesthesia in an operating room [2]. This chapter aims to demonstrate examples of difficulties during the implantation of the balloon and to suggest alternatives to solve these problems.

Clinical Case 1

A 48-year-old woman without comorbidities but with a body mass index (BMI) of 30.5 kg/m² sought medical help for weight loss. The team decided on the treatment with an IGB for 6 months.

The team decided on the treatment with an IGB for 6 months.

With a body mass index (BMI) of 30.5 kg/m²

A 48-year-old woman without comorbidities but with a body mass index (BMI) of 30.5 kg/m² sought medical help for weight loss. The team decided on the treatment with an IGB for 6 months.

S. A. Barrichello Júnior
Department of Bariatric Endoscopy, Healthme Clinic, São Paulo, SP, Brazil
e-mail: sergio.barrichello@healthme.com.br

L. G. de Quadros (✉)
Department of Digestive Surgery, ABC Faculty of Medicine, Santo André, SP, Brazil

© Springer Nature Switzerland AG 2020
M. Galvao Neto et al. (eds.), *Intragastric Balloon for Weight Management*,
https://doi.org/10.1007/978-3-030-27897-7_25

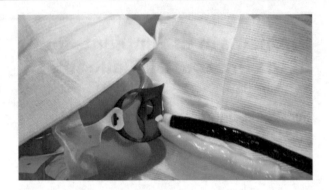

Fig. 25.1 Insertion of the device with a polypectomy snare, which holds the tip of the balloon before the introduction of the endoscope

Endoscopic Procedure

- An unsuccessful attempt to introduce the lubricated balloon was made, as the progression through the cricopharyngeal muscle could not be achieved.
- After the first attempt failed, a slight depression in the middle portion of the balloon was noticed. If the distal portion encountered resistance, it caused the device to kink and consequently lack stiffness to overcome minor obstacles.
- The passage of the balloon was succeeded using a polypectomy snare; before inserting it into the mouth, the snare was passed through the working channel and used to hold the balloon close to the distal tip (Fig. 25.1). The handle must be held in the applicator so that the balloon is not damaged. The device is gently driven through the cricopharyngeal muscle with to the endoscope, progressing to the stomach, where it is released. It is important to remember that the oral cavity offers a certain resistance as the balloon is passed over the scope.
- The remaining of the procedure occurred normally.

Clinical Case 2

A 30-year-old male with a BMI of 37.2 kg/m², with type 2 diabetes mellitus and arthralgia of the knees, sought medical help for weight loss. He refused bariatric surgery, therefore IGB treatment was indicated.

Endoscopic Procedure

- The balloon was introduced through the cricopharyngeal muscle uneventfully.
- After achieving the gastric chamber, the balloon started to progress roughly.
- As pressure was maintained on the catheter during the entrance in the gastric chamber, the greater curvature of the stomach obstructed the tip of the balloon precluding its progression and inflation (Fig. 25.2).

Fig. 25.2 Obstruction of the tip of the catheter in the greater curvature, precluding inflation of the balloon

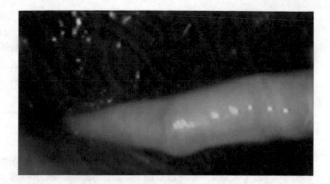

- The inflation catheter was pulled out a little to decrease the pressure at the tip of the balloon against the gastric wall.
- The IGB was guided to the adequate position using the endoscope or forceps (closed) as support.
- The anatomical landmarks were visualized to ensure inflation in a safe position inside the stomach.

Clinical Case 3

A 32-year-old woman with a body mass index (BMI) of 34.9 kg/m^2 and sleep obstructive apnea sought help for weight loss. She presented a shortened neck and a minor retrognathism. As she refused surgery, the implantation of an IGB for 6 months was indicated.

Endoscopic Procedure

- Some difficulty was found during the first attempt to insert the IGB.
- The endoscope was introduced to evaluate the positioning of the device; the balloon was twisted around the hypopharynx (Fig. 25.3).

Fig. 25.3 Image of the balloon twisted into the hypopharynx

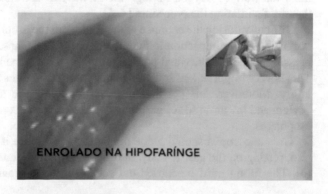

ENROLADO NA HIPOFARÍNGE

- The IGB was retracted and insertion was tried using the technique of chin lift to rectify the pharynx, thereby creating a more linear route. The fingers were used to properly position the balloon until it passed the pyriform sinus.
- After overcoming this obstacle, a slight pressure was applied, allowing the balloon to reach the stomach without further difficulties.

Discussion

Possible problems during balloon placement may be related to the positioning of the patient; the patient should be in the left lateral decubitus position, as perpendicular as possible to the bed if the airway is not protected during the procedure. In this position, the saliva tends to fall from the mouth instead of going to the larynx, which would cause cough and preclude the balloon passage [3].

Supporting the head of the patient to align the larynx makes the passage of the balloon smooth and less traumatic. During its introduction, the IGB touches the hypopharynx and the device is guided toward a pyriform sinus with a continuous pressure. If this route is not followed properly, an alternative is to guide the balloon using the index finger. Passage through the larynx under endoscopic control avoids unintentional insertion into the trachea.

Lubrication may facilitate the introduction of the balloon into the esophagus. Consequently, some manufacturers apply a lyophilized sheet over the device that becomes slippery in contact with saliva, thus facilitating its passage through the cricopharyngeal muscle. Introduction of the IGB should be smooth without any hasty maneuvers.

Small hiatal hernias, tortuosity of the esophagus, and extrinsic physiological constrictions may cause some difficulty in passing the IGB. Caution and care are essential to overcome such situations without lacerations, bleeding, and perforations. The introduction of the balloon with the aid of a polypectomy snare is an alternative; however, if further progression of the IGB is not easy under endoscopic control, we recommend the endoscopist to remove the device and retry, since insisting may cause injury.

For patients with micrognathia, the jaw thrust maneuver may be useful to optimize the flow of oxygen through the airway, in addition to aligning the larynx, thereby facilitating the procedure [4, 5].

Difficulty during the entrance of the IGB from the esophagus to the stomach may occur due to the impaction in the greater curvature. Thus, it may preclude its progression while the proximal portion remains in the lumen of the distal esophagus. This is very important, as inflation under these conditions may result in esophageal injury. Moreover, this positioning does not allow the adequate inflation of the device, and the air used for gastric distention escapes from the stomach toward the esophagus.

The endoscopist should guide the balloon and place it along the greater curvature, resting on the gastric body, in order to be under complete endoscopic control [6]. The filling must be carried out according to the manufacturer's instructions, respecting the material and volume of the device. The endoscopist must exchange the IGB immediately in case of any defects or leaks. After filling with the adequate volume and positioning according to the routine of the service, the valve must be disconnected. This step is central and the assistant physician should traction the catheter very gently since the resistance of the cardia is responsible for the detachment. If this resistance is greater than customary, a manufacturing defect should be suspected. At this time, caution is necessary. Twisting with the catheter or using the endoscope may assist the disconnection. If all these maneuvers fail to detach the balloon from the catheter, the safest option is to perforate the balloon, empty it, and exchange it for a new one.

In conclusion, technical precision and control of possible difficulties are needed in order to make the procedure safe and comfortable for the patient.

Final Considerations

- The implantation technique varies according to the type of balloon used.
- The procedure is safe and effective but requires specific training and care.
- Adequate tools should be available for IGB procedures.

References

1. Mathus-Vliegen EM, Alders PR, Chuttani R, et al. Outcomes of intragastric balloon placements in a private practice setting. Endoscopy. 2015;47(4):302–7.
2. Dabrowiecki S, Szczesny W, Poplawski C, et al. Intragastric Balloon (BIB system) in the treatment of obesity and preparation of patients for surgery – own experience and literature review. Pol Przegl Chir. 2011;83(4):181–7.
3. Gibson PG, Simpson JL, Ryan NM, et al. Mechanisms of cough. Curr Opin Allergy Clin Immunol. 2014;14(1):55–61.
4. Davies JD, Costa BK, Asciutto AJ. Approaches to manual ventilation. Respir Care. 2014;59(6):810–22; discussion 22–4.
5. Wysocki J, Krasny M, Prus M. Morphological predictors of sleep apnoea severity. Folia Morphol. 2016;75:107–11.
6. Gleysteen JJ. A history of intragastric balloons. Surg Obes Relat Dis. 2016;12(2):430–5.

Part V

Chronic Complications and Treatment

Helicobacter pylori and Intragastric Balloons

26

Felipe Matz Vieira and Flávio Mitidieri Ramos

Introduction

In 1983, in Australia, Marshall and Warren first identified the bacterium *Helicobacter Pylori* (*H. Pylori*), a discovery that led to the 2005 Nobel Prize in Medicine and Physiology. Since then, numerous human studies have identified it in different parts of the world and with different prevalence, varying from 8.7% to 85.5% [1–4]. Factors such as economic development, ethnicity, gender, and age may explain the different prevalence observed.

In general, it is estimated that more than half of the world's population is contaminated; however, only a tiny portion of the population will develop clinical diseases such as ulcer in the stomach or duodenum, or even gastric cancer. It is now recognized that more than 95% of the ulcers are caused by this bacterium and that its treatment can permanently cure the ulcer, preventing further crisis or complications. In relation to gastric cancer, the bacterium acts as an important risk factor for its development and is therefore considered by the World Health Organization to be a type 1 carcinogen for stomach cancer (in the same way as tobacco for lung cancer) [2]. Advances in public health, especially in basic sanitation, as well as in the general living conditions of the entire population have been associated with a progressive decrease in the prevalence of *H. Pylori* in the last 20 years [5–7].

The presence of *H. Pylori* in the mucosa of the stomach induces a chronic inflammatory process (gastritis), a scenario produced by the predominance of antibodies and cytokines induced by Th1 cells, which does not eliminate the pathogen, but favors a toxic environment for host cells. The rate of proliferation of gastric epithelial cells from *H. Pylori* infected patients is significantly higher than that of uninfected individuals. The continuous inflammatory process associated with high rates of cell turnover induces mutations, favoring the development of gastric cancer.

F. M. Vieira (✉) · F. M. Ramos
Department of Bariatric Endoscopy, Endodiagnostic, Rio de Janeiro, RJ, Brazil

© Springer Nature Switzerland AG 2020
M. Galvao Neto et al. (eds.), *Intragastric Balloon for Weight Management*,
https://doi.org/10.1007/978-3-030-27897-7_26

Helicobacter Pylori and Obesity

The prevalence of *H. Pylori* in obese individuals is not different from that observed in the general population, 8.7%, 53%, 85.5%, and 57% in Germany, Brazil, Saudi Arabia, and Colombia, respectively. However, there is still no consensus in the literature about the relationship between *H. Pylori* prevalence among obese and nonobese individuals. Epidemiological studies published in the last decade point to a relationship between the presence of *H. Pylori* and obesity, signaling that colonization could affect body mass index (BMI), but with inconsistent results [8–16].

Chronic gastritis induced by the presence of *H. Pylori* affects the regulation of gastric hormones, including ghrelin and leptin, both with significant roles in energy regulation. Thus, some authors state that there is a direct relationship between the absence of *H. Pylori* and weight gain. Among the probable explanations for this association is the fact that bacterial eradication would lead to increased gastric secretion of ghrelin, inducing increased appetite and consequently weight gain, and that eradication of the bacterium would also lead to a decreased expression of gastric leptin, accompanied by an increase in BMI [10–13]. However, two recently published studies did not corroborate such evidence [9, 17].

Reports of complications involving the use of the intragastric balloon (IGB) for the treatment of obesity and the presence of *H. Pylori* are scarce [18]. This can be explained in part by the fact that this method is effective and safe presenting complication rates close to zero, and adverse events such as obstruction, perforation, and death have an incidence of 0.3%, 0.1%, and 0.08%, respectively.

Anatomical alterations directly associated with *IGB* use are scarce, and there are no studies showing the relationship between anatomical changes and *H. Pylori*. However, it is known that the presence of the balloon in the stomach can lead to an increase in the thickness of the wall of the gastric body by increasing the thickness of the muscular layer, but this change is temporary and returns to baseline immediately after removal.

Diagnosis

Identification of the bacteria in the stomach can be performed during an endoscopy or by non-endoscopic methods. At endoscopy, it is detected by indirect methods (urea test) or by the presence of the bacteria in the tissue (histological investigation). Although not commonly used (due to the difficulties of its accomplishment), one can also try to cultivate the bacterium in small fragments obtained by biopsy of the stomach. In the case of endoscopic examination, five specimens should be collected, two from the antrum, two from the body, and one from the angularis *incisura* [19].

The presence of *H. Pylori* in the stomach can also be diagnosed without the aid of endoscopy. One of the most important and used methods is the labeled urea breath test, which is performed by collecting patient-breathed air into a collection bag, after ingesting a glass of orange juice mixed with carbon-13 labeled urea, a substance without smell, without taste, and harmless to health. It is an extremely effective test for diagnosis; in special situations, it is possible to detect the presence of *H. Pylori* through presence in blood and feces.

Treatment

Treatment is now recommended only in special situations, that is, routine testing is not recommended [8, 19]. Thus, all patients with an ulcer in the stomach and duodenum and infected by the bacteria should be treated. Likewise, first-degree relatives of people with stomach cancer should be investigated for the presence of the bacteria and, if so, submit to treatment. In other clinical situations, at the discretion of the physician, treatment may also be recommended.

The current treatment for bacterial elimination is based on the association of two antimicrobials and an antisecretory medication, administered during seven to ten days, with excellent results. The most indicated schedules are:

(a) Proton-pump inhibitor (PPI) in standard dose + amoxicillin 1.0 g + clarithromycin 500 mg twice daily for 7 days
(b) PPI at standard dose once daily + clarithromycin 500 mg twice daily + furazolidone 200 mg twice daily for 7 days
(c) PPI at standard dose once daily + furazolidone 200 mg three times a day + tetracycline hydrochloride 500 mg four times a day for 7 days [19, 20].

Unfortunately, the indiscriminate use of antibiotics has led to the emergence of strains of *H. Pylori* resistant to the usual treatment, requiring the use of alternative and potentially more toxic treatments.

Due to the alteration in gastric fundus pressure receptors, whose repercussions are delayed gastric emptying and consequent accumulation of gastric acid, it is inherent to the treatment of patients with the IGB device the routine use of PPI. Therefore, only in the presence of gastric lesions should the presence of *H. Pylori* be sought, and if so, initiate one of the treatment regimens recommended by the guidelines [19, 20].

One point that deserves attention is in relation to patients who use tobacco and who will be submitted to the treatment of obesity by the use of IGB. It is known that tobacco promotes changes in the gastric mucosa, and the cases of gastritis for gastric ulcers or even carcinoma can progress. In addition, smokers have a higher risk of being infected with *H. Pylori*, interfering negatively with the immune system [21].

For an infection with such dissemination index in the population, the ideal treatment would be the development of an anti-*H. Pylori* vaccine, administered in childhood. Although several biotechnology groups in different parts of the world have dedicated themselves to this task, the human results are still incipient, with a few years to be achieved.

References

1. Chang SS, Hu HY. Helicobacter pylori: effect of coexisting diseases and update on treatment regimens. World J Gastrointest Pharmacol Ther. 2015;6(4):127–36.
2. Hooi JKY, Lai WY, Ng WK, Suen MMY, Underwood FE, Tanyingoh D, et al. Global prevalence of Helicobacter pylori infection: systematic review and meta-analysis. Gastroenterology. 2017;153(2):420–9.
3. Ozdemir SH, Aksu C, Ozden E, Narman I, Varlik S, Aksu B, et al. Helicobacter pylori prevalence and relation with obesity. Indian J Pathol Microbiol. 2017;60(3):451–2.
4. Sugano K, Hiroi S, Yamaoka Y. Prevalence of Helicobacter pylori infection in Asia: remembrance of things past? Gastroenterology. 2018;154(1):257–8.
5. Araujo MB, Borini P, Guimaraes RC. Etiopathogenesis of peptic ulcer: back to the past? Arq Gastroenterol. 2014;51(2):155–61.
6. Khedmat H, Karbasi-Afshar R, Agah S, Taheri S. Helicobacter pylori infection in the general population: a Middle Eastern perspective. Caspian J Intern Med. 2013;4(4):745–53.
7. Malaty HM, Kim JG, Kim SD, Graham DY. Prevalence of Helicobacter pylori infection in Korean children: inverse relation to socioeconomic status despite a uniformly high prevalence in adults. Am J Epidemiol. 1996;143(3):257–62.
8. Wu MS, Lee WJ, Wang HH, Huang SP, Lin JT. A case-control study of association of Helicobacter pylori infection with morbid obesity in Taiwan. Arch Intern Med. 2005;165(13):1552–5.
9. Xu MY, Liu L, Yuan BS, Yin J, Lu QB. Association of obesity with Helicobacter pylori infection: a retrospective study. World J Gastroenterol. 2017;23(15):2750–6.
10. Tatsuguchi A, Miyake K, Gudis K, Futagami S, Tsukui T, Wada K, et al. Effect of Helicobacter pylori infection on ghrelin expression in human gastric mucosa. Am J Gastroenterol. 2004;99(11):2121–7.
11. Osawa H, Nakazato M, Date Y, Kita H, Ohnishi H, Ueno H, et al. Impaired production of gastric ghrelin in chronic gastritis associated with Helicobacter pylori. J Clin Endocrinol Metab. 2005;90(1):10–6.
12. Azuma T, Suto H, Ito Y, Ohtani M, Dojo M, Kuriyama M, et al. Gastric leptin and Helicobacter pylori infection. Gut. 2001;49(3):324–9.
13. Nishi Y, Isomoto H, Uotani S, Wen CY, Shikuwa S, Ohnita K, et al. Enhanced production of leptin in gastric fundic mucosa with Helicobacter pylori infection. World J Gastroenterol. 2005;11(5):695–9.
14. Kawano S, Kawahara A, Nakai R, Fu HY, Tsuji S, Tsujii M. Helicobacter pylori infection does not affect serum leptin concentration and body mass index (BMI) in asymptomatic subjects. J Gastroenterol. 2001;36(8):579–80.
15. Lane JA, Murray LJ, Harvey IM, Donovan JL, Nair P, Harvey RF. Randomised clinical trial: Helicobacter pylori eradication is associated with a significantly increased body mass index in a placebo-controlled study. Aliment Pharmacol Ther. 2011;33(8):922–9.
16. Yang YJ, Sheu BS, Yang HB, Lu CC, Chuang CC. Eradication of Helicobacter pylori increases childhood growth and serum acylated ghrelin levels. World J Gastroenterol. 2012;18(21):2674–81.
17. den Hollander WJ, Broer L, Schurmann C, Meyre D, den Hoed CM, Mayerle J, et al. Helicobacter pylori colonization and obesity – a Mendelian randomization study. Sci Rep. 2017;7(1):14467.
18. Yoo IK, Chun HJ, Jeen YT. Gastric perforation caused by an intragastric balloon: endoscopic findings. Clin Endosc. 2017;50(6):602–4.
19. Coelho LG, Maguinilk I, Zaterka S, Parente JM, do Carmo Friche Passos M, Moraes-Filho JP. 3rd Brazilian consensus on Helicobacter pylori. Arq Gastroenterol. 2013;50(2):81.
20. Sheu BS, Wu MS, Chiu CT, Lo JC, Wu DC, Liou JM, et al. Consensus on the clinical management, screening-to-treat, and surveillance of Helicobacter pylori infection to improve gastric cancer control on a nationwide scale. Helicobacter. 2017;22(3):e12368.
21. Koivisto TT, Voutilainen ME, Farkkila MA. Effect of smoking on gastric histology in Helicobacter pylori-positive gastritis. Scand J Gastroenterol. 2008;43(10):1177–83.

Fungal Colonization

27

Artagnan Menezes Barbosa de Amorim,
Victor Ramos Mussa Dib,
and Manoel Galvao Neto

Introduction

Obesity is one of the worse diseases of the humanity. Treatment options consist of calorie-restricted diet, lifestyle modification, medical treatment, endoscopic IGB insertion, endoscopic gastroplasty, and bariatric surgery. The IGB was based on the observation that long-lasting and well-tolerated gastric bezoars can result in significant weight loss. It acts as an artificial bezoar, in theory, delays gastric emptying, and maintains the feeling of satiety for longer [1]. IGB therapy, as part of a multidisciplinary weight management program, is an effective short-term intervention for weight loss.

The IGB can be indicated for patients with overweight and obesity refractory to behavioral and medical treatment to achieve a weight loss of at least 10% of the original weight or 25% of overweight. It is indicated for patients with BMI higher or equal than 27 kg/m^2 and obese class III patients (BMI > 40 kg/m^2) who hesitate to undergo surgery despite having criteria for treatment with bariatric surgery [2].

A. M. B. de Amorim (✉)
Department of Endoscopy, 9 de Julho Hospital, São Paulo, SP, Brazil

V. R. M. Dib
Department of Surgery, Victor Dib Institute, Manaus, AM, Brazil

M. Galvao Neto
Department Digestive Surgery, ABC Faculty of Medicine, São Paulo, SP, Brazil

Department of Bariatric Endoscopy, Endovitta Institute, São Paulo, SP, Brazil

© Springer Nature Switzerland AG 2020
M. Galvao Neto et al. (eds.), *Intragastric Balloon for Weight Management*,
https://doi.org/10.1007/978-3-030-27897-7_27

Clinical and Diagnostic Aspects of the Disease

The more common complications of the IGB procedure are balloon intolerance, gastric ulcer, gastric erosion and esophagitis, spontaneous deflation of the balloon, ongoing vomiting for 1–3 weeks or more, abdominal pain, and gastroesophageal reflux [3]. There are also a few reported cases of gastric perforation and small intestinal obstruction. Infection arising from intragastric balloon insertion is not a common issue. In unusual situations, fungal colonization of the IGB is observed, sometimes on their content, a condition that is asymptomatic in most cases [2].

The fungal and bacterial colonization can occur on the surface of IGB presented as the result of different factors, which predisposes to opportunistic infections such as gastric stasis, smoking, and use of antacid drugs. Colonization is generally asymptomatic and occurs on the outer surface of the IGB. In most cases, it is discovered at the time of removal, sometimes altering the physical characteristics of the balloon, making it brittle and hardened, which can make removal more difficult [2]. Spontaneous deflation of the balloon may be a risk factor. This should be taken into consideration, especially in immunosuppressed patients who should be monitored. Any asymptomatic balloon infection should be treated, especially those with damaged gastrointestinal mucosa. When symptoms are present, they are nonspecific such as epigastric pain, vomiting, and, in severe cases, dysphagia [2].

Candida is a yeast and is the most common cause of opportunistic fungal infection worldwide. It is also a frequent colonizer of human skin and mucous membranes. *Candida* is a constituent of the normal flora of the skin, mouth, vagina, and stool. Colonization of soft lining materials with microorganisms, particularly *Candida* species, is a common clinical problem. The IGB has a silicon elastomer structure with soft lining materials that are more susceptible to *Candida* adhesion.

Candidiasis of the gastrointestinal system mostly affects the esophagus, with infection seen as patchy plaques on the mucosa. Fungal infection is usually not detected in the esophagus of patients elected to use IGB. Contamination cannot be excluded and may occur during endoscopic intervention, that is, the balloon passage through the oral cavity or during its insertion.

Delayed gastric emptying and gastric stasis have been proposed as predisposing factors causing gastric candidiasis. It is a well-known issue that one of the mechanisms of action of the IGB is to delay gastric emptying. Thus, the slowing down of normal peristalsis of the stomach by the IGB may allow opportunistic organisms to colonize more readily.

The patients in whom an IGB is inserted should take proton-pump inhibitors because of gastric hyperacidity. These proton-pump inhibitors result in a hypochlorhydric gastric medium, which makes opportunistic infections more likely.

When the infection on the balloon is a local colonization rather than systemic, we recommended appropriate nonspecific supportive treatment for the patient. However, systemic antifungal and antibacterial treatment are recommended for patients in whom the gastrointestinal integrity is damaged, who are immunocompromised or scheduled for bariatric surgery.

Case Reports

1. A 28-year-old woman, 124 kg in weight, and BMI 43.2 kg/m². During retrieval of the balloon, endoscopic findings were unremarkable, but the surface of the balloon was covered with necrotic green-white plaques (Fig. 27.1).
2. A 38-year-old obese female, 89.2 kg, BMI 35 kg/m², with many unsuccessful attempts at weight loss with dietary restriction and medications for about 2 years. After evaluation with the multidisciplinary team, a 1-year adjustable intragastric balloon (AIGB) was indicated.

After the initial period of adaptation, the patient showed a satisfactory evolution with loss of 12.3 kg (BMI 30 kg/m²) until the end of the second month of treatment when she started presenting epigastric pain, postprandial fullness, and vomiting. A computed tomography showed abnormal balloon inflation with air inside. The patient was submitted to an endoscopic evaluation that showed a visually hyperinflated balloon with marked fluid level with about 50% of the balloon with air (Fig. 27.2).

Fig. 27.1 Endoscopic view of IGB colonized with fungus, showing necrotic green-white plaques covering the surface of the device

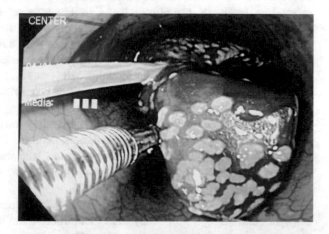

Fig. 27.2 Endoscopic view of a hyperinflated balloon, showing an air–fluid level

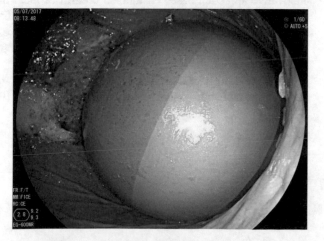

The management adopted was to completely empty the AIGB, with the first 50 mL sent for culture (which identified the presence of Candida sp.), followed by new insufflation with 10 mL of nystatin solution (1,000,000 units) added to 600 mL of methylene blue solution.

Follow-up was done with nutrition and endoscopy staff. A new tomography showed a correctly located balloon in gastric fundus and with no gas. There was no need of other interventions. After 6 months, the patient remained asymptomatic with current weight of 68 kg, weight loss so far of 19.5 kg, and BMI of 27.24 kg/m^2 (22.28% of initial weight). Removal was planned for 12 months [2].

Discussion

Nystatin is a polyene antifungal antibiotic obtained from *Streptomyces noursei* and its molecular formula is $C_{47}H_{75}NO_{17}$. Nystatin is both fungistatic and fungicidal in vitro against a wide variety of yeasts and yeast-like fungi. *Candida albicans* demonstrates no significant resistance to nystatin in vitro on repeated subculture in increasing levels of nystatin; other Candida species become quite resistant. Generally, resistance does not develop in vivo. Nystatin acts by binding to sterols in the cell membrane of susceptible Candida species with a resultant change in membrane permeability allowing leakage of intracellular components. Nystatin exhibits no appreciable activity against bacteria protozoa or viruses. Gastrointestinal absorption of nystatin is insignificant. Most orally administered nystatin is passed unchanged in the stool [2].

The contamination of the IGB and its content raises the possibility of gas production inside the balloon by fungal fermentation, resulting in increased diameter and balloon volume leading to obstructive symptoms (nausea, vomiting, ulcers, ischemia, and perforation). In these situations, typically the balloon is removed, and pharmacologic treatment is not necessary [2].

Marques et al. show that the choice for treating fungal contaminated IGB by emptying and filling it up with nystatin in addition to methylene blue solution is an innovative approach based on rational control of local infection. In some cases, it shows to be well succeeded by no recurrence of hyperinflation with gas. Despite the success of the approach in these cases, it still requires prospective randomized studies to confirm the effectiveness of the use of nystatin prophylaxis/treatment for fungal contamination in balloons that allow adjustment.

An algorithm for management of symptomatic and asymptomatic hyperinflation of 1-year adjustable intragastric balloon has been proposed (Fig. 27.3 – from Ref. [2]).

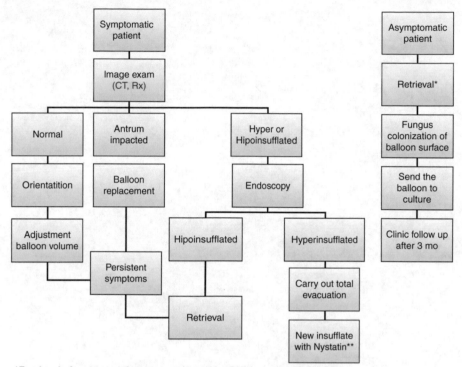

*Retrieval after 1 year of treatment; ** 10mL of Nistatin (1.000.000 ul)

Fig. 27.3 Proposed algorithm for management of colonized balloons [2]

References

1. Kotzampassi K, Vasilaki O, Stefanidou C, Grosomanidis V. Candida albicans colonization on an intragastric balloon. Asian J Endosc Surg. 2013;6(3):214–6.
2. Marques LM, Souza TF, Grecco E, Galvao Neto MP, Ramos FM, Vieira FM, Garcia VG, Freitas CE. Proposed treatment of adjustable intragastric balloon contaminated with Candida. Bariatric Surg Pract Patient care. 2015;10:169–72.
3. Simsek Z, Gurbuz OA, Coban S. Fungal colonization of intragastric balloons. Endoscopy. 2014;46(Suppl 1 UCTN):E642–3.

Part VI

Special Populations

Intragastric Balloons in Pediatric Patients and Special Populations

28

Manoel Galvao Neto, Lyz Bezerra Silva,
Luiz Gustavo de Quadros, Idiberto José Zotarelli Filho,
and Josemberg M. Campos

Introduction

In recent decades, the incidence and prevalence of childhood obesity has increased in most countries. According to the National Health and Nutrition Examination Surveys (NHANES) in the USA, the prevalence of obesity in children aged 6–11 years increased from 4.2% in the 1960s to 19.6% in 2007–2008, that is about a fivefold increase in 40 years [1, 2]. Moreover, in the adult population, the prevalence of the most relevant comorbidities, such as hypertension, type II diabetes, and metabolic syndrome, increased from 2.8% in 1980 to 6.4% in 2011, with an estimate of about 20% of the population being affected by 2021 [3–9]. In addition to this, obesity affects special populations, such as patients with total or partial *situs inversus*, the elderly and individuals with chronic diseases, thereby increasing comorbidities and making treatment more difficult [10].

M. Galvao Neto
Department Digestive Surgery, ABC Faculty of Medicine, São Paulo, SP, Brazil

Department of Bariatric Endoscopy, Endovitta Institute, São Paulo, SP, Brazil

L. B. Silva · J. M. Campos
Department of Surgery, Federal University of Pernambuco, Recife, PE, Brazil

L. G. de Quadros (✉)
Department of Digestive Surgery, ABC Faculty of Medicine, Santo André, SP, Brazil

I. J. Zotarelli Filho
Department of Endoscopy, Kaiser Clinic, São José do Rio Preto, São Paulo, Brazil

© Springer Nature Switzerland AG 2020
M. Galvao Neto et al. (eds.), *Intragastric Balloon for Weight Management*,
https://doi.org/10.1007/978-3-030-27897-7_28

Today, childhood obesity has a significant short- and long-term impact on children's health and well-being in both industrialized and developing countries [1, 11]. In the last two decades, according to the World Health Organization (WHO), childhood obesity has increased considerably worldwide [10]. Consequently, obese children are more prone to develop cardiac, pulmonary, psychological, and endocrine diseases, many of which persist into adulthood [11–14].

Thus, obese children are one of the main target groups for the application of strategies to prevent and control excess weight including obesity, not because of their characteristics as a risk group, but because of the chances of success [15–17]. The American Academy of Pediatrics (AAP) rates the body mass index (BMI) of children and adolescents by percentiles, considering the child to be overweight when values are between the 85th and 95th percentile. The AAP states that, over the past 30 years, the population of obese children in the United States has been increasing and now affects about 20% of the child population [18]. The age range between 5 and 7 years corresponds to one of the phases of greater susceptibility for the development of obesity. In this period, the BMI increases rapidly after a period of reduced adiposity so that fast and/or intense fat deposition at this stage may indicate an increased risk of obesity in the future [18].

The traditional clinical treatment for obesity in children and in special populations includes several types of interventions: low-calorie, low-sugar and high-protein diets, and changes in the family's daily life [19]. However, these treatments tend to fail in the case of patients with severe obesity and metabolic issues. In this setting, in which the available therapies have limited and non-lasting results, the use of an intragastric balloon (IGB) is recognized as an effective treatment with a long-lasting result, especially in patients with delicate profiles [20].

In addition to bariatric endoscopy in children, the implantation of an IGB is a technique used before bariatric surgery or as a single procedure in patients who do not want surgery or who are at high operative risk. The use of an IGB is also strongly indicated for special patients with chronic diseases, the elderly and individuals with *situs inversus*, because it is less invasive and traumatic [21–23]. However, it is necessary to increase the number of prospective randomized studies to confirm and optimize the benefits of IGB use in these types of patients [24–36].

Thus, the present chapter sought to gather the most important published information on the use of IGBs in obese children and special patients in order to assist readers in decision-making about the use of this device for safe and effective weight loss.

Discussion

Intragastric Balloons in Pediatric Patients

The International Pediatric Endosurgery Group (IPEG) published a series of guidelines proposing to perform bariatric procedures, including endoscopy to implant IGBs, in children with a BMI greater than 35 kg/m² associated with type II diabetes, moderate obstructive sleep apnea or pseudotumor cerebri, or a BMI greater than 40 kg/m^2 even without comorbidities. Additional criteria for such procedures include bone maturity of 95.0% or more, demonstrated commitment to change lifestyle, and stable psychosocial environment [14]. In addition, the patient should clearly understand the associated implications through a clarification process that culminates in the legal guardian's signature of an informed consent form, a document in which information on risks, benefits, and responsibilities must be well defined [15].

Despite this IPEG's proposal, pediatric procedures are controversial because of the immediate risks of surgery and the ethical implications and long-term complications associated with this procedure. Moreover, there is uncertainty about the efficacy of this operation since this patient profile may not be able to follow the diet and make the lifestyle changes necessary to maintain the success of the procedure in the postoperative period [14].

In addition, both the short- and long-term response of patients submitted to IGB placement aimed at restoring their health and well-being is still unknown [18]. Given the scarcity of information, it is very difficult to construct a risk--benefit profile as to the child's therapeutic response to any of the restrictive or malabsorptive surgical procedures. Beneficence also supports the inclusion of low-risk children in clinical trials with validated tests that allow weight loss using medications [18]. Furthermore, studies addressing the topic of bariatric procedures in cases of obesity in children show that there is no consensus in respect to this population [18–20]. One cannot overlook the fact that children and adolescents are in full development and therefore subject to changes in their bodies [24, 25, 37–39].

As literature background, the board of the Spanish Society for the Surgery of Obesity and Metabolic Disorders (SECO) proposed a study of childhood obesity using the Delphi method. This prospective study involved 60 experts from nine national societies. Each society recruited specialists in fields related to obesity [19]. Two online questionnaires were used, and a consensus on the guidelines of several treatments for obesity was reached according to the percentages of favorable and unfavorable responses for the inclusion of each guidelines. The results of the study indicated significant concern of all the societies regarding obesity. There was a strong consensus regarding pediatric obesity, medical treatment, dietary recommendations, environmental and social factors, and goals for obese children [19].

Consensus on the use of IGBs and other techniques was not achieved. However, biliopancreatic diversion was rejected as primary treatment, and a mandatory psychological/psychiatric evaluation was agreed upon. Accepted inclusion criteria were similar to those of adults with the exception of surgery in those with a BMI <40 Kg/m^2. Spanish societies connected to obesity are aware of the social problem of childhood obesity. The multisocial development of national approaches may arise from consensus studies by specialists [19].

Another study evaluated the efficacy of a new IGB for the treatment of morbidly obese children [12]. Obalon®(Obalon Therapeutics Inc., Carlsbad, CA, USA) was first used in 17 obese children in order to assess its safety and efficacy in reducing excess weight. In 9 of the 17 children, a second balloon was placed 30–40 days after the first insertion. All the IGBs were removed by endoscopy after an average of 18 weeks. In the group of 16 patients who completed the study (one patient was still under treatment), the mean weight decreased from 95.8 ± 18.4 to 83.6 ± 27.1 kg ($p < 0.05$) and the mean BMI decreased from 35.27 ± 5.89 (range: 30.4–48) to 32.25 ± 7.1 kg/m^2 (range: 23.5–45.7) ($p > 0,05$); the mean excess weight, calculated according to the Cole curves for pediatric populations, decreased from 36.2 ± 15.9 to 29.4 ± 18.3 kg ($p = 0.14$) with a percentage excess weight lost of 20.1 ± 9.8 (range: 2.3–35.1). The waist circumference decreased from 109 ± 12.3 to 99 ± 10.5 cm ($p < 0.05$). Therefore, Obalon® can be administered easily without complications, inducing significant weight loss with a statistically significant reduction in BMI and an improvement in associated comorbidities [12].

According to de Peppo et al. [12], different types of IGBs have been used in pediatric and adolescent patients with varying degrees of obesity. The most widely used is the BioEnterics®IGB (BIB – Allergan, Irvine, CA). The complications of the BIB were gastric ulcers, gastric erosions, esophagitis, spontaneous deflation, persistent vomiting, gastroesophageal reflux, and pain. There are also some reports of gastric perforations, small intestinal obstructions, and significant gastric dilatation.

Given these concerns, the Obalon® device was developed; in most cases (82%), patients were able to swallow the device without sedation, and general anesthesia was required only at the end of the treatment with the removal of the IGB. Moreover, the Obalon® device can be used from a lower threshold BMI (>30 Kg/m^2) compared to the BIB and other IGBs because of its reduced side effects and complication rates. These aspects make this device safe in young patients with moderate obesity with or without comorbidities.

After a thorough review of the preliminary results, de Peppo et al. [12] decided to treat only patients with Class I obesity with BMI between 30 and 35 Kg/m^2. The results obtained in this study confirm the efficacy of the treatment in these children. Thus, patients were included in the study despite having BMIs that were lower than the value recommended by the European Guidelines on severe obesity surgery [40].

Therefore, the results of this study demonstrated that the Obalon® device can be easily implanted without anesthesia in most patients (83%) and induces significant weight loss within 3 months. The use of the Obalon® device for more than 13 weeks, as suggested by the manufacturer, resulted in spontaneous deflation in three patients and unnoticed spontaneous expelling of the balloon in two of the three patients. Despite this, the device can be considered a useful tool for the management of subjects with Class I obesity and guarantee an appreciable weight loss, particularly in children and adolescents with BMI <35 Kg/m^2 [12].

Nobili et al. [13] also evaluated the efficacy of the Obalon®IGB on weight loss and in respect to metabolic and cardiovascular parameters in ten pediatric patients with severe obesity. All patients were submitted to anthropometric evaluations, biochemical tests, ultrasound examinations of the liver, and blood pressure monitoring at the time of insertion and removal of the device. The Obalon®IGB had a positive effect on weight loss, BMI, and percentage of excess body weight lost within 3 months. In addition, this minimally invasive device improves the cardiometabolic profiles of obese children.

Special Populations – The Elderly, Chronic Diseases, and *Situs Inversus*

The use of IGBs was investigated in the context of metabolic syndrome. One study analyzed the effect of 6 months treatment on the health-related quality of life (HRQoL) of patients and in relation to changes in body fat in obese individuals with metabolic syndrome [18]. Fifty 18- to 50-year-old obese patients with metabolic syndrome were selected for 6 months of treatment. Body fat was assessed using anthropometric parameters and dual energy radiological absorptiometry (DXA) at the beginning of treatment and immediately after removing the IGB.

The HRQoL was also assessed using the abbreviated World Health Organization Quality of Life questionnaire (WHOQOL-BREF) at the beginning and shortly after IGB removal. Thirty-nine patients completed the study. After 6 months, there was a significant improvement in the perceptions of quality of life ($p = 0.0009$), health ($p < 0.0001$), and in the physical ($p = 0.001$), psychological ($p = 0.031$), and environmental domains ($p = 0.0071$). The anthropometric measurements and total fat determined by DXA were directly and significantly related to an improvement in the general aspects of quality of life [18]. The decrease in the percentage of total fat was the parameter that best correlated with improvements in the perception of quality of life ($p = 0.032$). Hence, in obese individuals with metabolic syndrome, weight loss parameters were associated with short-term improvements in HRQoL after 6 months of IGB treatment. However, only total fat was independently correlated to the perception of HRQoL [18].

Obesity is a serious disease with increasing incidence among over 60-year-old individuals [41]. Thus, IGB treatment can reduce the BMI by 5–9 kg/m^2 over 6 months, with an impressive improvement in obesity-related comorbidities. In this context, a study was performed of 106 men (47.1%) and 119 women (52.9%) submitted to IGB placement. Of these, 12 patients (8 women and 4 men) were over 60 years of age. An average excess weight loss of 31.4 was recorded for the 12 elderly patients; two patients suffered severe esophagitis requiring removal of the IGB and one late gastric perforation was reported. A significantly higher complication rate ($p < 0.001$) was found for the elderly population compared to the other patients. Thus, IGB treatment is considered safe and effective for elderly patients in terms of weight loss and improvement in comorbidities even though IGB can cause complications that can sometimes be serious, such as esophageal trauma and gastric perforation. An in-depth instrumental study and a rigorous follow-up is advised in all cases of suspected complications [41].

These findings were also consistent with the study of the BioEnterics IGB® (BIB) and the Spatz® Adjustable Balloon System (Spatz Medical, Great Neck, NY, USA). Patients with ages ranging from 70 to 80 years and BMIs between 37 and 46 submitted to BIB implantation from January 2010 to July 2012 were retrospectively studied. Furthermore, a prospective study of a similar population of patients treated with the Spatz balloon was performed from July 2012 to August 2014 [42]. This study compared the two types of IGB in terms of weight loss, complications, and weight maintenance after removal. For both treatments, the median weight loss was

20 ± 3 kg and the median BMI at the end of therapy was 32 ± 2; no severe complications occurred [42].

Some studies are notable in relation to the use of IGBs in chronic diseases [18, 43, 44]. The results of IGB placement to achieve weight loss in obese patients with chronic kidney disease (CKD) were reported in a study that aimed to assess the safety and efficacy of IGBs as a weight loss treatment in this patient population [43]. A prospective, single-arm, "first-in-CKD" study was conducted in Stage 3–4 CKD patients with BMI >35 kg/m^2 referred for weight loss. After clinical evaluations, the IGB was inserted endoscopically in the stomach where it remained for 6 months. Complications, adverse events, acceptability, weight loss, and metabolic responses were monitored during this period. Eleven participants were recruited over 18 months. Nine patients completed the study and two patients withdrew (one before IGB implantation and one early withdrawal after three days due to persistent vomiting). There were five episodes of acute renal injury occurring in three patients [43].

Six months after implantation, the mean body mass had decreased by 9.6% (SD $\pm$ 6.8%). The median waist circumference and total cholesterol had decreased significantly [7.7 cm (interquartile range: 15.3–3.9) and 0.2 mmol/L (IQR: 0.6–0.05), respectively], with no significant change in the estimated glomerular filtration rate, blood pressure, triglycerides, adipocytokines, inflammation, or arterial stiffness as measured by carotid–femoral pulse wave velocity. On removal of the IGB, there was one case of gastritis and another of esophagitis. Therefore, treatment with IGBs has only moderate efficacy in weight loss with a high complication rate in obese patients with established CKD [43].

Also, in the context of chronic diseases, endoscopic IGB placement can be used as a minimally invasive technique to promote weight loss and reduce the risks in liver transplant candidates. In one study, liver transplant candidates with a BMI >40 kg/m^2 or a BMI between 35 and 40 and a low graft-to-weight ratio were considered for weight reduction [44]. IGBs were implanted in six men and two women with a mean age of 46 ± 5 years and a mean BMI of 43.5 ± 6.9 kg/m^2. All patients except one with hepatocellular carcinoma had decompensated liver disease with a mean Child score of 8.5 ± 1.6. All patients had transient vomiting except one, in which balloon volume was decreased due to persistent vomiting. All but one patient had weight loss and none of the patients had serious complications. Liver transplantation was successful in five (three deceased and two liver transplants from living donors) patients all of whom had a post-transplant course without complications after weight loss while three patients were still waiting for donors. Moreover, three of the five patients maintained the weight loss after transplantation. Therefore, IGB placement is a useful modality to promote short-term weight loss and render morbid obese recipients fit for liver transplant surgery [44].

The use of IGB has been reported in a super-obese patient with *situs inversus totalis* and asymptomatic cholelithiasis who underwent endoscopic IGB placement in preparation for bariatric surgery. Subsequently, laparoscopic cholecystectomy and adjustable laparoscopic gastric banding were performed in the same session. Special attention was given to reviewing the literature and modifying the specular image of laparoscopic cholecystectomy and laparoscopic gastric banding procedures. The operation can be performed safely with preoperative evaluations and modifications in the surgical team and equipment [45].

Final Considerations

The use of endoscopic devices has been reported for many years in respect to the challenges against obesity and comorbidities in pediatric and special populations, with most results being positive. Therefore, the IGB is an important tool for bariatric endoscopy in high-risk surgical patients.

References

1. Tauber M. Obesity and overweight of children and adolescents. Rev Prat. 2015;65:1263.
2. Wang Y, Lobstein T. Worldwide trends in childhood overweight and obesity. Int J Pediatr Obes. 2006;1:11–25.
3. Kelishadi R. Childhood overweight, obesity, and the metabolic syndrome in developing countries. Epidemiol Rev. 2007;29:62–76.
4. Skoczen S, Wojcik M, Fijorek K, et al. Expression of the central obesity and type 2 diabetes mellitus genes is associated with insulin resistance in young obese children. Exp Clin Endocrinol Diabetes. 2015;123:252–9.
5. Mondini L, Levy RB, Saldiva SRDM, Venâncio SI, Aguiar JA, Stefanini MLR. Prevalência de sobrepeso e fatores associados em crianças ingressantes no ensino fundamental em um município da região metropolitana de São Paulo, Brasil. CadSaúdePública(RiodeJaneiro).ago. 2007;23(8):1825–34.
6. Ogden CL, Flegal KM. Changes in terminology for childhood overweight and obesity. Natl Health Stat Rep. 2010;25:1–5.
7. Weiss R, Dziura J, Burgert TS, Tamborlane WV, Taksali SE, Yeckel CW, et al. Obesity and the metabolic syndrome in children and adolescents. N Engl J Med. 2004;350(23):2362–74.
8. Carvalho MA, Carmo I, Breda J, Rito AI. Análise comparatva de métodos de abordagem da obesidade infantl. Rev Port Saúde Pública. 2011;29(2):148–56.
9. Levine MD, Ringham RM, Kalarchian MA, Wisniewski L, Marcus MD. Is family-based behavioral weight control appropriate for severe pediatric obesity? Int J Eat Disord. 2001;30(3):318–28.
10. Aikenhead A, Knai C, Lobstein T. Do surgical interventons to treat obesity in children and adolescents have long- versus short-term advantages and are they cost-effectve? HEN synthesis report june 2012. [Internet]. Copenhagen: WHO Regional Office for Europa; 2012 [acesso 25 jan 2014]. Disponível: http://www.euro.who.int/__data/assets/pdf_fle/0009/165825/e96550.pdf.
11. Sachdev P, Reece L, Thomson M, Natarajan A, Copeland RJ, Wales JK, Wright NP. Intragastric balloon as an adjunct to lifestyle programme in severely obese adolescents: impact on biomedical outcomes and skeletal health. Int J Obes (Lond). 2018;42(1):115–8. https://doi.org/10.1038/ijo.2017.215. Epub 2017 Sep 5.
12. De Peppo F, Caccamo R, Adorisio O, Ceriati E, Marchetti P, Contursi A, Alterio A, Della Corte C, Manco M, Nobili V. The Obalonswallowable intragastric balloon in pediatric and adolescent morbid obesity. Endosc Int Open. 2017;5(1):E59–63. https://doi.org/10.1055/s-0042-120413.
13. Nobili V, Corte CD, Liccardo D, Mosca A, Caccamo R, Morino GS, Alterio A, De Peppo F. Obalon intragastric balloon in the treatment of paediatric obesity: a pilot study. Pediatr Obes. 2015;10(5):e1–4. https://doi.org/10.1111/ijpo.268. Epub 2014 Nov 14.

14. Palermo TM, Dowd JB. Childhood obesity and human capital accumulation. Soc Sci Med. 2012;75(11):1989–98.
15. Prat JS, Lenders CM, Dionne EA, Hoppin AG, Hsu GL, Inge TH, et al. Best practice updates for pediatric/adolescent weight loss surgery. Obesity (Silver Spring). 2009;17(5):901–10.
16. Hofmann B. Bariatric surgery for obese children and adolescents: a review of the moral challenges. BMC Med Ethics. [Internet]; 2013 [acesso 5 mar 2015];14:18. Disponível: http://www.biomedcentral.com/1472-6939/14/18.
17. Tomicic JT, Luks FI, Shalon L, Tracy TF. Laparoscopic gastrostomy in infants and children. Eur J Pediatr Surg. 2002;12(2):107–10.
18. Guedes EP, Madeira E, Mafort TT, Madeira M, Moreira RO, de Mendonça LMC, de Godoy-Matos AF, Lopes AJ, Farias MLF. Impact of 6 months of treatment with intragastric balloon on body fat and quality of life in obese individuals with metabolic syndrome. Health Qual Life Outcomes. 2017;15(1):211. https://doi.org/10.1186/s12955-017-0790-x.
19. Vilallonga R, Moreno Villares JM, Yeste Fernández D, Sánchez Santos R, Casanueva Freijo F, Santolaya Ochando F, Leal Hernando N, Lecube Torelló A, Castaño González LA, Feliu A, Lopez-Nava G, Frutos D, de la Cruz Vigo F, Torres Garcia AJ, Ruiz de Adana JC. Initial approach to childhood obesity in Spain. A multisociety expert panel assessment. Obes Surg. 2017;27(4):997–1006. https://doi.org/10.1007/s11695-016-2413-8.
20. Rahman AA, Loi K. Gastric Perforation as a complication of intragastric balloon. Surg Obes Relat Dis. 2018;pii: S1550–7289(18):30034. https://doi.org/10.1016/j.soard.2018.01.019.
21. Leeman MF, Ward C, Duxbury M, de Beaux AC, Tulloh B. The intra-gastric balloon for pre-operative weight loss in bariatric surgery: is it worthwhile? Obes Surg. 2013;23(8):1262–5. https://doi.org/10.1007/s11695-013-0896-0.
22. Moura D, Oliveira J, De Moura EG, et al. Effectiveness of intragastric balloon for obesity: a systematic review and meta-analysis based on randomized control trials. Surg Obes Relat Dis. 2016;12(2):420–9.
23. Kumar N. Endoscopic therapy for weight loss: gastroplasty, duodenal sleeves, intragastric balloons, and aspiration. World J Gastrointest Endosc. 2015;7(9):847–59.
24. Borges AC, Almeida PC, Furlani SMT, Cury MS, Gaur S. Intragastric balloons in high-risk obese patients in a Brazilian center: initial experience. Rev Col Bras Cir. 2018;45(1):e1448. https://doi.org/10.1590/0100-6991e-20181448. Epub 2018 Feb 15.
25. Alsabah S, Al Haddad E, Ekrouf S, Almulla A, Al-Subaie S, Al Kendari M. The safety and efficacy of the procedureless intragastric balloon. Surg Obes Relat Dis. 2018;14(3):311–7. https://doi.org/10.1016/j.soard.2017.12.001. Epub 2017 Dec 9.
26. Kumar N, Bazerbachi F, Rustagi T, McCarty TR, Thompson CC, Galvao Neto MP, Zundel N, Wilson EB, Gostout CJ, Abu Dayyeh BK. The influence of the orberaintragastric balloon filling volumes on weight loss, tolerability, and adverse events: a systematic review and meta-analysis. Obes Surg. 2017;27:2272–8.
27. Ponce J, Woodman G, Swain J, et al. The Reduce pivotal trial: a prospective, randomized controlled pivotal trial of a dual intragastric balloon for the treatment of obesity. Surg Obes Relat Dis. 2015;11:874–81.
28. Laing P, Pham T, Taylor LJ, et al. Filling the void: a review of intragastric balloons for obesity. Dig Dis Sci. 2017;62(6):1399–408.
29. IBGE- Instituto Brasileiro de Geografia e Estatística. Disponível em: http://www.ibge.gov.br. Acesso em março de 2016.
30. Mathus-Vliegen EM, Alders PR, Chuttani R, Scherpenisse J. Outcomes of intragastric balloon placements in a private practice setting. Endoscopy. 2015;47(4):302–7.
31. Nobili V, Corte CD, Liccardo D, et al. Obalonintragastric balloon in the treatment of paediatric obesity: a pilot study. Pediatr Obes. 2015;10:e1–4.
32. Genco A, Bruni T, Doldi SB, et al. BioEnterics intragastric balloon: the Italian experience with 2,515 patients. Obes Surg. 2005;15:1161–4.
33. Brooks JI, Srivastava ED, Mathus-Vliegen EM. One-year adjustable intragastric balloons: results in 73 consecutive patients in the U. K. Obes Surg. 2014;24:813–9.

34. Genco A, Dellepiane D, Baglio G, et al. Adjustable intragastric balloon vs non-adjustable intragastric balloon: case-control study on complications, tolerance, and efficacy. Obes Surg. 2013;23:953–8.
35. De Peppo F, Di Giorgio G, Germani M, et al. BioEntericsintragastric balloon for treatment of morbid obesity in Prader-Willi syndrome: specific risks and benefits. Obes Surg. 2008;18:1443–9.
36. Kirby DF, Wade JB, Mills PR, et al. A prospective assessment of the Garren-Edwards Gastric Bubble and bariatric surgery in the treatment of morbid obesity. Am Surg. 1990;56:575–80.
37. FDA Recently-apprived devices. Obalon System—P160001. Center for Devices and Radiological Health. http://www.fda.gov/medicaldevices/productsandmedicalprocedures/deviceapprovalsandclearances/recently-approveddevices/ucm520741.htm. Accessed 12 Dec 2017.
38. Abu Dayyeh BK. Intragastric balloons for obesity management. Gastroenterol Hepatol (NY). 2017;13(12):737–9.
39. Tate CM, Geliebter A. Intragastric balloon treatment for obesity: FDA safety updates. Adv Ther. 2018;35(1):1–4. https://doi.org/10.1007/s12325-017-0647-z. Epub 2017 Dec 28.
40. Fried M, Yumuk V, Oppert JM, et al. Interdisciplinary European guidelines on metabolic and bariatric surgery. Obes Surg. 2014;24:42–55.
41. Velotti N, Bianco P, Bocchetti A, Milone M, Manzolillo D, Maietta P, Amato M, Buonomo O, Petrella G, Musella M. Acute complications following endoscopic intragastric balloon insertion for treatment of morbid obesity in elderly patients. A single center experience. Minerva Chir. 2018. https://doi.org/10.23736/S0026-4733.18.07712-X.
42. Russo T, Aprea G, Formisano C, Ruggiero S, Quarto G, Serra R, Massa G, Sivero L. BioEnterics intragastric balloon (BIB) versus spatz adjustable balloon system (ABS): our experience in the elderly. Int J Surg. 2017;38:138–40. https://doi.org/10.1016/j.ijsu.2016.06.013. Epub 2016 Jun 21.
43. MacLaughlin HL, Macdougall IC, Hall WL, Dew T, Mantzoukis K, Oben JA. Does intragastric balloon treatment for obesity in chronic kidney disease heighten acute kidney injury risk? Am J Nephrol. 2016;44(6):411–8. Epub 2016 Oct 27.
44. Choudhary NS, Puri R, Saraf N, Saigal S, Kumar N, Rai R, Rastogi A, Goja S, Bhangui P, Ramchandra SK, Raut V, Sud R, Soin A. Intragastric balloon as a novel modality for weight loss in patients with cirrhosis and morbid obesity awaiting liver transplantation. Indian J Gastroenterol. 2016;35(2):113–6. https://doi.org/10.1007/s12664-016-0643-2. Epub 2016 Apr 13.
45. Taskin M, Zengin K, Ozben V. Concomitant laparoscopic adjustable gastric banding and laparoscopic cholecystectomy in a super-obese patient with situsinversustotalis who previously underwent intragastric balloon placement. Obes Surg. 2009;19(12):1724–6. https://doi.org/10.1007/s11695-008-9725-2.

Intragastric Balloons as a Bridge to Bariatric and Non-bariatric Surgery in Super-Obese Patients

29

Manoel Galvao Neto, Lyz Bezerra Silva, Luiz Gustavo de Quadros, Idiberto José Zotarelli Filho, and Josemberg M. Campos

Introduction

In some cases, the surgical treatment of super-obese patients (body mass index – BMI >50 kg/m²) is impossible due to unacceptable risk. Ideally, it is recommended that patients should lose at least 10% of their total weight in order to diminish the risks and postoperative complications [1]. However, a large proportion of super-obese patients are unable to lose weight on diets alone and require other methods to achieve this goal. In this context, intragastric balloon (IGB) placement is a technique used before bariatric surgery, or even as an isolated procedure in patients who do not want to undergo surgery. Moreover, IGBs are used as a bridge to surgery in super-obese patients who have high operative risk [1, 2].

Super obesity is associated with various comorbidities such as diabetes, hypertension, and cardiovascular disease [3]. A weight loss of 5–10% may be

M. Galvao Neto
Department Digestive Surgery, ABC Faculty of Medicine, São Paulo, SP, Brazil

Department of Bariatric Endoscopy, Endovitta Institute, São Paulo, SP, Brazil

L. B. Silva · J. M. Campos
Department of Surgery, Federal University of Pernambuco, Recife, PE, Brazil

L. G. de Quadros (✉)
Department of Digestive Surgery, ABC Faculty of Medicine, Santo André, SP, Brazil

I. J. Zotarelli Filho
Department of Endoscopy, Kaiser Clinic, São José do Rio Preto, São Paulo, Brazil

© Springer Nature Switzerland AG 2020
M. Galvao Neto et al. (eds.), *Intragastric Balloon for Weight Management*,
https://doi.org/10.1007/978-3-030-27897-7_29

enough to delay or prevent the onset of these comorbidities, however, the availability of safe and effective weight loss therapies is limited [4, 5]. Bariatric surgery is the most effective treatment in combating this chronic complex disease, nevertheless it is a high-risk surgical procedure due to the severity of the obesity in these individuals [5, 6].

Preoperative treatment with an IGB significantly reduces liver volume in super-obese patients, thereby facilitating Roux-en-Y bypass surgery [1, 7]. However, because its mechanism of weight loss is mostly restrictive, its efficacy largely depends on the patient's adherence to lifestyle changes (diet and exercise). On average, this method allows a total weight loss of 12.0–15.0% [8].

Thus, the IGB is an effective and feasible bridge to surgery that should be considered when faced with difficulties due to enlarged livers in patients with a high BMI who are indicated for sleeve gastrectomy [9]. The goal of the IGB is to reduce both the liver size and visceral fat efficiently, thereby facilitating the bariatric procedure [9]. However, further prospective randomized studies are necessary to confirm these benefits.

Thus, the present chapter aims to collect the main data on the use of IGBs in super-obese patients.

Discussion

Super obesity is considered a nutritional disorder; more common in Western countries and is correlated to high morbidity and mortality [1–4]. Different approaches are used in the treatment of obesity, including diet, behavioral therapy, medications, and surgery [3, 4]. If patients do not meet the criteria for bariatric surgery or are at high surgical risk, IGBs can be employed to reduce weight prior to the procedure. Currently, the IGB is one possible bariatric technique used to treat super-obese patients [1–6].

The placement of IGBs is increasingly being employed as an option for the treatment of obesity in patients with BMI >27 kg/m^2 in Europe and Brazil or >30 kg/m^2 in the United States when they fail to control their weight with diet and exercise. IGBs are also being used in patients who lack the criteria for or refuse weight reduction surgery, and as a bridge to surgery in super obesity when the BMI $\geq$50 kg/m^2 [6, 7]. In super-obese patients, preoperative treatment with an IGB significantly reduces liver volume to facilitate the Roux-en-Y bypass surgery [7].

A randomized study compared the use of an IGB for 6 months with standard medical care after which laparoscopic gastric bypass was performed. IGB insertion for 6 months before gastric bypass was efficient at inducing weight loss [3].

Patients with high BMIs (>60 kg/m^2) are at a greater postoperative risk and difficulties are commonly encountered during surgery [13]. Studies have shown that outcomes are optimized with a multidisciplinary approach toward the management of these patients that prioritizes patient safety [14]. In respect to this, the use of an IGB has the advantage of being minimally invasive [15].

A meta-analysis comparing the effectiveness of the IGB and diet shows that the IGB technique provides a greater likelihood of weight loss [15]. Furthermore, one study showed that operative complications, duration of surgery, and postoperative complications were reduced in patients who underwent IGB placement prior to surgery [16, 17]. This could allow less invasive methods to be used in super-obese patients with fewer side effects as well as decreasing the need for hospitalization. In addition, hepatic steatosis was diminished from 52% to 4% in patients who achieved reductions in weight with the insertion of an IGB [18].

Other studies have shown that IGBs were cost-effective and reduced postoperative mortality when used as a bridge to bariatric surgery [19, 20]. Mortality is especially high in super-obesity as the patient is at increased risk of life due to the possibility of laceration when the left liver lobe is lifted. Studies have found that the insertion of an IGB is effective to reduce liver size and consequently prevent this type of complication [21].

Many studies have demonstrated the efficacy of IGBs for short-term weight loss in obese and super-obese patients with significant reductions in comorbidities [1–7, 22–26]. Due to the increase in their use and the lack of standardization of the technique, a consensus meeting was organized involving endoscopists and surgeons with high volumes of IGB cases [27]. The objective of the meeting was to discuss and evaluate the procedural aspects of IGBs (indications, contraindications, technique, management of complications, etc.); a consensus was reached on the best practices based on the scientific literature and expert experience [28, 33, 34]. In addition, the Brazilian statistics were presented, highlighting the country's significant experience with this procedure [32, 36, 39].

The South Pacific has a high prevalence of obesity and super-obesity. A retrospective review of a laparoscopy database for sleeve gastrectomy examined 494 patients, 46 of whom had previously received an IGB. The mean initial BMI was 47.8 kg/m^2. For all patients who received the IGB, the subsequent bariatric procedure was successful [4]. Another study with 20 super-obese patients showed that preoperative weight loss is important to reduce surgical risk. Hospitalization and low-calorie diets are safe and effective. The rate of weight loss stabilized 14 weeks after the insertion of an IGB signaling the time for the surgical intervention [5].

A study conducted by Leeman et al. [6] analyzed 28 super-obese patients with BMIs >55 kg/m^2 who received IGBs ($n = 15$) or not ($n = 13$) to assist in weight loss prior to bariatric surgery. The objective was to achieve a 10% excess weight loss in 6 months. Only two patients in the IGB group and three in the non-IGB group failed to reach the goal. Although the comparative analysis did not present any significant difference, the use of the balloon facilitated the bariatric procedure.

Another study retrospectively evaluated the results of patients receiving IGBs over 3 years. It was found that the IGB is an effective temporary option to treat morbid obesity. However, careful patient selection and good monitoring by the surgical department are very important so that the results can be optimized [8]. One case-controlled study compared the records of 60 consecutive super-super-obese patients (BMI: >66.5 ± 3.4 kg/m^2) submitted to laparoscopic vertical gastrectomy. IGB prior to surgery significantly reduced excess BMI, which was also associated with a shorter surgical time and lower overall risks of significant adverse complications [10].

A retrospective study by Gottig et al. [11] evaluated the safety and efficacy of IGBs in obese patients. The mean weight loss at the time of balloon removal was 21.2 ± 14.0 kg. The mean BMI loss and excess BMI loss were 7.2 kg/m^2 and 30.1 kg/m^2, respectively. Of the 190 patients, 76 performed surgery (40%). Of these, seven patients had a BMI <50 kg/m^2, while all other patients were super-obese (BMI >50 kg/m^2). Furthermore, 58 patients (30.5%) who had a BMI >60 kg/m^2 and presented a high surgical risk were able to undergo surgery due to substantial weight loss and/or reduced comorbidities with the use of the IGB. Thus, IGB has been shown to be a safe, tolerable, and effective procedure for the initial treatment of morbid obesity.

Spyropoulos et al. [13] found that the placement of an IGB can be considered an effective first-stage treatment in high-risk, super-obese patients requiring surgical interventions. Although not without risk, it is usually a simple procedure that leads to satisfactory weight loss, amelioration of comorbidities and consequent reduction of mortality rates, and perioperative morbidity associated with the surgery.

A meta-analysis that evaluated balloons filled with saline and methylene blue with volumes ranging from 400 to 700 mL enrolled more than 2000 super-obese patients. This study found a decrease in BMI by 9 kg/m^2 after 6 months of use [10]. In addition to weight loss, improvements in blood pressure, fasting blood glucose, and the lipid profile were also observed. Significant decreases or normalization of glycated hemoglobin levels were reported in 87.2% of the patients [16].

In addition to weight loss, the IGB has a significant metabolic effect, especially in super-obese individuals, with a decrease in the prevalence of hyperglycemia from 50% to 12% and hypertriglyceridemia from 58% to 19% [7, 10]. Depression also improved in 70.8% of cases with a significant decrease in the prevalence of severe depression from 27.7% to 1.5% [17].

A recent systematic review with meta-analysis analyzed nine randomized studies involving air- or liquid-filled balloons with volumes between 400 and 900 mL. This study demonstrated that IGB use in comparison to just diet gave better results in terms of final weight (weight loss: 3.55 kg; 95% confidence interval: 6.20–0.90) and BMI (decrease in BMI: 2.62 kg/m^2; 95% confidence interval: 4.92–0.33) [12]. In addition, quantitative analysis showed a statistically significant difference in favor of the IGB group for the percentual loss of excess weight (14%; p-value <0.005). Furthermore, an evaluation performed 5 years after the removal of the IGB found a mean weight loss of 7.3 ± 5.4 kg and a decrease in BMI of 2.5 kg/m^2 with the values in the 6-month evaluation being 23.9 ± 9.1 kg and 8.3 kg/m^2, respectively [18].

Another study evaluated short-term efficacy, tolerance, and complications in high-risk super-obese patients treated with IGB as a bridge to surgery. A *post hoc* analysis was conducted at a Brazilian university hospital from 2010 to 2014 of 23 adult patients with a mean BMI of 48 kg/m^2 who received a single air- or liquid-filled IGB [20]. Efficacy was defined as a 10% loss of excess weight and complications were defined as adverse events related to the IGB diagnosed after the initial adaptation period. The balloons, the majority (65.2%) air-filled, were effective in 91.3% of the patients, remaining in situ for an average of 5.5 months. The mean weight loss was 23.7 ± 9.7 kg (loss of excessive weight $21.7\% \pm 8.9$) and mean BMI reduction was 8.3 ± 3.3 kg/m^2. Complications were reported in 17.3% of the cases and included abdominal discomfort, balloon deflation, and delayed intolerance, but without severe difficulties; the majority of participants (82.7%) had no adverse effects. The IGBs were removed at the correct time without intercurrences and 52.2% of these patients underwent bariatric surgery 1 month after removal. Therefore, IGBs can be successfully used as an initial weight-loss procedure, with good tolerance and acceptable complication rates [20].

The Elipse® Balloon (Allurion Technologies Inc., Natick, MA, USA) is a new balloon design that managed to get around some difficulties, but research on its effectiveness is important. Thus, a prospective multicenter study examined the use of the Elipse® Balloon in super-obese patients [40]. The weight, BMI, and occurrence of adverse events were documented over 4 months. One hundred and thirty-five patients with a mean age of 33.5 years were enrolled in the study. At 4 months, the mean weight loss of the patients was 13.0 kg (p-value $= 0.000$) and the mean BMI decreased by 4.9 kg/m^2 (p-value $= 0.000$). The mean total weight loss was 15.1%. All patients reported nausea on the first day of insertion; however, 69.6% reported complete resolution by Day 3. Two (1.5%) patients had vomited the balloon early, three (2.2%) patients had the balloon removed early due to intolerance, three patients (2.2%) had early deflation, 18 (13.3%) patients reported episodes of diarrhea around the time of deflation, and 29 (21.5%) patients presented abdominal pain with colic during the week the balloon was deflated. One patient presented obstruction of the small intestine after which the balloon was removed by laparoscopic enterotomy. Thus, the Elipse® Balloon effectively aided weight loss with promising results [40].

In addition, the presence of IGB may lead to an increase in the thickness of the gastric body wall due to hypertrophy of its muscular layer. These changes are apparently transitory, 30 days after the removal of the balloon the wall thickness returned to the values observed before IGB placement [39]. However, thickening of the gastric wall caused by the presence of the balloon may increase the risk of leaks [39].

Even though most of the literary findings show the viability of the IGB as a bridge to bariatric surgery, the technique exposes the patient to general anesthesia three times – during balloon insertion and removal and during the surgery itself [29–31, 35, 37, 38]. In addition, the IGB increases the chance of having increased gastric wall tension, and technically subsequent stapling can expose the patient to complications; the patient should wait for a certain period for the wall of the stomach to return to its normal size [9, 40].

Final Considerations

The use of endoscopic devices has been reported for many years, reducing the challenges to treat super obesity and its comorbidities with positive results for most patients. Therefore, the IGB is an important tool in the treatment of super-obese patients who have elevated surgical risk for gastroplasty. IGB is an effective and feasible bridge to surgery that should be considered when faced with difficulties due to an enlarged liver in patients with high BMIs who are indicated for vertical gastrectomy.

References

1. Keren D, Rainis T. Intragastric balloons for overweight populations-1 year post removal. Obes Surg. 2018;28:2368. https://doi.org/10.1007/s11695-018-3167-2.
2. Rahman AA, Loi K. Gastric Perforation as a complication of intragastric balloon. Surg Obes Relat Dis. 2018;14(5):719–22. https://doi.org/10.1016/j.soard.2018.01.019.
3. Coffin B, Maunoury V, Pattou F, Hébuterne X, Schneider S, Coupaye M, Ledoux S, Iglicki F, Mion F, Robert M, Disse E, Escourrou J, Tuyeras G, Le Roux Y, Arvieux C, Pouderoux P, Huten N, Alfaiate T, Hajage D, Msika S. Impact of intragastric balloon before laparoscopic gastric bypass on patients with super obesity: a randomized multicenter study. Obes Surg. 2017;27(4):902–9. https://doi.org/10.1007/s11695-016-2383-x.
4. Lemaître F, Léger P, Nedelcu M, Nocca D. Laparoscopic sleeve gastrectomy in the South Pacific. Retrospective evaluation of 510 patients in a single institution. Int J Surg. 2016;30:1–6. https://doi.org/10.1016/j.ijsu.2016.04.002.
5. Santo MA, Riccioppo D, Pajecki D, Rd C, Kawamoto F, Cecconello I. Preoperative weight loss in super-obese patients: study of the rate of weight loss and its effects on surgical morbidity. Clinics (Sao Paulo). 2014;69(12):828–34. https://doi.org/10.6061/clinics/2014(12)07.
6. Leeman MF, Ward C, Duxbury M, de Beaux AC, Tulloh B. The intra-gastric balloon for preoperative weight loss in bariatric surgery: is it worthwhile? Obes Surg. 2013;23(8):1262–5. https://doi.org/10.1007/s11695-013-0896-0.
7. Frutos MD, Morales MD, Lujan J, Hernández Q, Valero G, Parrilla P. Intragastric balloon reduces liver volume in super-obese patients, facilitating subsequent laparoscopic gastric bypass. Obes Surg. 2007;17(2):150–4.
8. Carvalho MR, Jorge Z, Nobre E, Dias T, Cortez-Pinto H, Machado MV, Camolas J, Neves S, Guerra A, Vieira J, Fagundes MJ, Brito MJ, Almeida Nunes P, do Carmo I. Intra-gastric ballon in the treatment of morbid obesity. Acta Medica Port. 2011;24(4):489–98.. Epub 2011 Dec 12
9. Al-Sabah S, Al-Marri F, Vaz JD. Intragastric balloon as a bridge procedure in patients with high body mass index. Surg Obes Relat Dis. 2016;12(10):1900–1. https://doi.org/10.1016/j.soard.2016.08.494.
10. Zerrweck C, Maunoury V, Caiazzo R, Branche J, Dezfoulian G, Bulois P, Verkindt H, Pigeyre M, Arnalsteen L, Pattou F. Preoperative weight loss with intragastric balloon decreases the risk of significant adverse outcomes of laparoscopic gastric bypass in super-super obese patients. Obes Surg. 2012;22(5):777–82. https://doi.org/10.1007/s11695-011-0571-2.
11. Göttig S, Weiner RA, Daskalakis M. Preoperative weight reduction using the intragastric balloon. Obes Facts. 2009;2(Suppl 1):20–3. https://doi.org/10.1159/000198243.
12. Frutos MD, Morales MD, Luján J, Hernández Q, Valero G, Parrilla P. Intragastric balloon reduces liver volume in super-obese patients, facilitating subsequent laparoscopic gastric bypass. Obes Surg. 2007;17(2):150–4.
13. Spyropoulos C, Katsakoulis E, Mead N, Vagenas K, Kalfarentzos F. Intragastric balloon for high-risk super-obese patients: a prospective analysis of efficacy. Surg Obes Relat Dis. 2007;3(1):78–83.
14. Kakarla VR, Nandipati K, Lalla M, Castro A, Merola S. Are laparoscopic bariatric procedures safe in superobese (BMI Z50 kg/m^2) patients? AnNSQIP data analysis. Surg Obes Relat Dis. 2011;7(4):452–8.
15. Orlando G, Gervasi R. Luppinol etal. Theroleofa multidisciplinary approach in the choice of the best surgery approach in a super-super-obesity case. Int J Surg. 2014;12(Suppl1):S103–6.

16. Moura D, Oliveira J, De Moura EG, et al. Effectiveness of intragastric balloon for obesity: a systematic review and meta-analysis based on randomized control trials. Surg Obes Relat Dis. 2016;12(2):420–9.
17. Forlano R, Ippolito AM, Iacobellis A, et al. Effect of the BioEnterics intragastric balloon on weight, insulin resistance, and liver steatosis in obese patients. Gastrointest Endosc. 2010;71(6):927–33.
18. Majumder S, Birk J. Are view of the current status of endoluminal therapy as a primary approach to obesity management. Surg Endosc. 2013;27(7):2305–11.
19. Kumar N. Endoscopic therapy for weight loss: gastroplasty, duodenal sleeves, intragastric balloons, and aspiration. World J Gastrointest Endosc. 2015;7(9):847–59.
20. Borges AC, Almeida PC, Furlani SMT, Cury MS, Gaur S. Intragastric balloons in high-risk obese patients in a Brazilian center: initial experience. Rev Col Bras Cir. 2018;45(1):e1448. https://doi.org/10.1590/0100-6991e-20181448. Epub 2018 Feb 15
21. FDA   Recently-ApprivedDevices.Obalon   System—P160001.   Center   for   Devices   and Radiological   Health.   http://www.fda.gov/medicaldevices/productsandmedicalprocedures/deviceapprovalsandclearances/recently-approveddevices/ucm520741.htm. Accessed 12 Dec 2017.
22. Inc., Apollo Endosurgery. Orbera TM intragastric balloon system (Orbera TM). San Diego: Apollo Endosurgery; 2015. p. 1–30.
23. Abu Dayyeh BK. Intragastric balloons for obesity management. Gastroenterol Hepatol (N Y). 2017;13(12):737–9.
24. Alsabah S, Al Haddad E, Ekrouf S, Almulla A, Al-Subaie S, Al Kendari M. The safety and efficacy of the procedureless intragastric balloon. Surg Obes Relat Dis. 2018;14(3):311–7. https://doi.org/10.1016/j.soard.2017.12.001. Epub 2017. Dec 9
25. Barham K, Dayyeh A. Intragastric balloons for obesity management. Gastroenterol Hepatol (N Y). 2017;13(12):737–9.
26. Tate CM, Geliebter A. Intragastric balloon treatment for obesity: FDA safety updates. Adv Ther. 2018;35(1):1–4. https://doi.org/10.1007/s12325-017-0647-z.. Epub 2017 Dec 28
27. Kumar N, Bazerbachi F, Rustagi T, McCarty TR, Thompson CC, Galvao Neto MP, Zundel N, Wilson EB, Gostout CJ, Abu Dayyeh BK. The influence of the orberaintragastric balloon filling volumes on weight loss, tolerability, and adverse events: a systematic review and meta-analysis. Obes Surg. 2017;12:2272–8.
28. Almeghaiseeb ES, Ashraf MF, Alamro RA, et al. Efficacy of intragastric balloon on weight reduction: Saudi perspective. World J Clin Cases. 2017;5(4):140–7.
29. Yorke E, Switzer NJ, Reso A, et al. Intragastric balloon for management of severe obesity: a systematic review. Obes Surg. 2016;26(9):2248–54.
30. Ponce J, Woodman G, Swain J, et al. The reduce pivotal trial: a prospective, randomized controlled pivotal trial of a dual intragastric balloon for the treatment of obesity. Surg Obes Relat Dis. 2015;11:874–81.
31. Laing P, Pham T, Taylor LJ, et al. Filling the void: a review of intragastric balloons for obesity. Dig Dis Sci. 2017;62(6):1399–408.
32. IBGE- Instituto Brasileiro de Geografia e Estatística. Disponível em: http://www.ibge.gov.br. Acessoemmmarço de 2016.
33. Miranda da Rocha LC, Ayub Perez OA, Arantes V. Endoscopic management of bariatric surgery complications: what the gastroenterologist should know. Rev Gastroenterol Mex. 2016;81(1):35–47.
34. Mathus-Vliegen EM, Alders PR, Chuttani R, Scherpenisse J. Outcomes of intragastric balloon placements in a private practice setting. Endoscopy. 2015;47(4):302–7.
35. Lecumberri E, Krekshi W, Matía P, Hermida C, de la Torre NG, Cabrerizo L, Rubio MÁ. Effectiveness and safety of air-filled balloon Heliosphere BAG® in 82 consecutive obese patients. Obes Surg. 2011;21(10):1508–12.
36. Galvao Neto M, Marins Campos J. Therapeutic flexible endoscopy after bariatric surgery: a solution for complex clinical scenarios. Cir Esp. 2015;93(1):1–3.

37. Angrisani L, Santonicola A, Iovino P, Formisano G, Buchwald H, Scopinaro N. Bariatric surgery worldwide. Obes Surg. 2015;25(10):1822–32.
38. Malik VS, Willett WC, Hu FB. Global obesity: trends, risk factors and policy implications. Nat Rev Endocrinol. 2013;9(1):13–27.
39. Périssé LGS, Périssé PCM, Ribeiro KF. Gastric wall changes after intragastric balloon placement: a preliminary experience. Rev Col Bras Cir. 2016;43(4):286–8.
40. Alsabah S, Al Haddad E, Ekrouf S, Almulla A, Al-Subaie S, Al Kendari M. The safety and efficacy of the procedureless intragastric balloon. Surg Obes Relat Dis. 2018;14(3):311–7. https://doi.org/10.1016/j.soard.2017.12.001. Epub 2017. Dec 9

Part VII

Miscellaneous

Drug Regimen and Intragastric Balloon: Pre, Post, During, Combined

30

Elaine Moreira and Antonio Fábio Teixeira

Introduction

The predominance of obesity worldwide has nearly doubled since 1980, with current estimates of 2.1 billion affected individuals. Overweight and obesity lead to numerous adverse conditions, including type 2 diabetes, cardiovascular disease, stroke, and certain types of cancer. The global spread of obesity and comorbidities not only threatens the quality of life, but also represents a significant economic burden [1].

Although bariatric surgery has proven to be a viable treatment option for the morbidly obese, there is clearly a need for less invasive alternatives.

The use of associated drugs during the treatment with the intragastric balloon (IGB) is a very broad subject, of great importance, and, at the same time, with little scientific basis. Didactically, we have divided this chapter in two sections:

- Drug use for symptoms relief, which occur frequently in the period after IGB placement. These can be used before, during, or after the procedure. Also, medications used to prevent possible complications from the prosthesis are addressed.
- Antiobesity drugs, which can be used as concomitant to the IGB or after its removal in order to enhance weight loss and help in maintaining it.

E. Moreira (✉)
Department of Bariatric Endoscopy and Gastroenterology, Endovitta Institute, São Paulo, SP, Brazil

A. F. Teixeira
Department of Surgery and Physiology, Gastros Bahia, Feira de Santana, BA, Brazil

© Springer Nature Switzerland AG 2020
M. Galvao Neto et al. (eds.), *Intragastric Balloon for Weight Management*,
https://doi.org/10.1007/978-3-030-27897-7_30

Medications for IGB Symptoms Relief

Drugs Before Balloon Placement

Some professionals use medications before balloon placement with the intent to relieve abdominal discomfort and, mainly, nausea and vomiting immediately after the procedure. The most commonly used drugs in this phase are steroids, antiemetics, antispasmodic, and proton-pump inhibitors (PPIs). [2]

As there are not enough evidences that the use of these medications with a preventive action significantly changes the clinical symptoms during or immediately after intragastric balloon placement, this practice is not a mandatory step.

Drugs Used During IGB Placement

In addition to the anesthetics, during the implant procedure, intravenous medications can be used for relief of symptoms that are common and appear already in the early hours after the procedure [2].

Usually these are antiemetic, analgesic, and antiacid drugs with the intention of reducing the common symptoms in the first few days after placement, for example, aprepitant, ondansetron, ranitidine, intravenous omeprazole.

This is also not a mandatory conduct. However, the routine use of intravenous infusion of symptomatic medications relieves the common adverse events in the early post-placement period of IGB.

Drugs Used After IGB Placement

After IGB placement, when the patient is discharged, the oral use of symptomatic medication should be initiated in order to reduce the discomfort and common symptoms. The most commonly used drugs are listed in Table 30.1:

Table 30.1 Drugs used during and after the procedure of intragastric balloon

Symptoms	Drugs	Drug administration	Comments
Nausea	Chloridrate of metoclopramide	Oral (oral solution and tablet) Intramuscular Intravenous	Should not be used in epileptic patients Side effects: Drowsiness, restlessness, extrapyramidal symptoms, depression, diarrhea Risk of malignant neuroleptic syndrome (MNS)
	Ondansetrone	Oral (sublingual) Intravenous	5-HT3 receptor antagonist Sublingual - may be ingested without water
	Dimenidrinate	Oral (oral solution, tablet and capsigel) Intramuscular Intravenous	Dimenhydrin + pyridoxine hydrochloride (tablet) = less side effects Common adverse effect: Drowsiness, dizziness, visual turbidity Capsigel: May be ingested without water Pharmacologically belongs to the class of antihistamines
	Aprepitant/Phosaprepitanto Dimeglumine	Oral Intravenous	80 mg or 125 mg tablets Injectable: Fosaprepitanto, dimeglumina May be administered in combination with ondansetron or dexamethasone, thus increasing the antiemetic effect Acts by centrally antagonizing receptors of the substance for neurokinin-1 Adverse effect: Fatigue, weakness, constipation, diarrhea, hiccups High cost
	Domperidone	Oral (oral suspension and tablet)	Is an antiemetic and gastroduodenal motor regulator that stimulates gastric peristalsis from the center, actively promoting emptying of the stomach May increase abdominal discomfort Also used for heartburn and regurgitation Common side effects: Depression, anxiety, headache, drowsiness, diarrhea, pruritus, asthenia

(continued)

Table 30.1 (continued)

Symptoms	Drugs	Drug administration	Comments
Abdominal pain and discomfort	Scopolamine butylbromide	Oral (oral solution, tablet and dram) Intramuscular Intravenous Subcutaneous	Anticholinergic substance, has strong hallucinogenic effects Side effects: Dry mouth, dilated pupils, dry throat, cessation of saliva production, nasal mucosae and urinary retention Contraindicated in the elderly
	Tramadol	Oral (oral solution, tablet and capsule) Intramuscular Intravenous Subcutaneous	Centrally acting opioid analgesic Moderate to severe pain Common adverse effects: Headache, drowsiness, vomiting, constipation, dry mouth, perspiration fatigue
Heartburn	PPIs Omeprazole *20 mg or 40 mg* Esomeprazole *20 mg or 40 mg* Lansoprazole *15 mg or 30 mg* Pantoprazole *20 mg or 40 mg* Dexlansoprazole *30 mg or 60 mg*	Oral (tablet and capsule) Intravenous	Decrease the acidity of the stomach through inhibition of the proton pump Injectables: Pantoprazole sodium 40 mg Medications indicated for continuous use throughout the duration of the balloon in the stomach

Source: Brazilian Intragastric Balloon Consensus Statement – BIBC (2018) [3]

It is worth remembering that the drugs mentioned above can be used during the entire period of intragastric balloon treatment, in case of any symptoms presented by the patient.

Antiobesity Drugs During IGB Treatment

The treatment strategy for obesity has undergone profound changes in recent years. The rational use of antiobesity drugs is currently considered an indispensable adjunct to many obese patients when there is already a great risk to health. The definition criteria for its use have always been a major concern. Consensus statements are unanimous in recommending that pharmacotherapy should always be used in conjunction with a patient lifestyle change program [4].

In the face of the antiobesity drugs in association with the intragastric balloon, the most used with satisfactory results, safety, and reduced adverse effects is liraglutide.

The daily dose of liraglutide can reach 3.0 mg, being marketed under the brand name Saxenda® and has recently been approved by the Food and Drug Administration (FDA) and the European Medicine Agency (EMA) as adjuvant of a comprehensive lifestyle intervention to achieve weight loss [5].

Studies have shown that liraglutide treatment in addition to weight reduction has also induced a decrease in waist circumference, serum triglycerides, insulin resistance, blood pressure, and an increase in high-density lipoprotein cholesterol (HDL-C). The most common side effects were nausea, hypoglycemia, diarrhea, constipation, vomiting, and headache [6].

In the treatment of obesity, regardless of the technique used, it is necessary to modify habits, with a healthy diet and regular physical exercise [7]. Especially when using the IGB, the patient should be supported, guided, and encouraged by follow-up with an interdisciplinary team during the period in which the balloon remains in place.

Discussion

Clinical Treatment of Obesity

Obesity is associated with several comorbid conditions, such as diabetes mellitus, dyslipidemia, hypertension, coronary artery disease, sleep apnea, osteoarticular diseases, and some types of cancer. In view of its multicasuality, a multidisciplinary approach is necessary in its treatment. The use of drugs in the treatment of obesity still suffers nowadays an unfounded and prejudiced resistance, both by clinicians and patients, in view of the erroneous concept of risk of dependence and addiction associated with these drugs, usually related to amphetamines [8] (Table 30.2).

Table 30.2 Weight loss drugs

Medication	Dose/day
Phentermine	37.5 mg
Topiramate	100 mg
Qsymia	15 mg/92 mg
Belviq	20 mg
+Contrave	32 mg/160 mg
Xenical	360 mg
Saxenda	3.0 mg

Source: Camilleri (2018) [9]

Amphetamine-derived anorectic agents, which are now used, have little potential for dependence and, in general, a low financial cost. Thus, we consider the combination of several techniques and concepts in the therapy of excess weight reasonable.

Anorectic and lipolytic femproporex together with the application of concepts and practices of cognitive behavioral therapy showed good results in the treatment of obesity [10]. This is a low-cost drug that can be used by a large population: an effective drug, with few side effects and toxicity, low potential for dependence, and low pharmacological tolerance.

Recently, several evidences indicate that obesity is associated with a subclinical inflammatory process. The importance of recognizing obesity as an inflammatory state is due to the possibility that inflammation is one of the links between obesity and insulin resistance, systemic arterial hypertension, and cardiovascular disease [11]. Therefore, the use of antioxidant medications has been shown to be efficient in the clinical control of obesity. Several studies have shown that weight loss is associated with decreased insulin resistance and inflammatory markers.

Phytotherapy emerges as another low-cost alternative and few side effects in the treatment of obesity [12]. With a possible weight-loss effect, it should be prescribed and monitored in the same way as allopathic medication, since it does not have proven safety and efficacy. *Camelia sinesis* was confirmed as a promoter of weight reduction by stimulation of lipid oxidation and thermogenesis [13].

It is known that obesity is a chronic disease where there is an important cause-and-effect relationship with intestinal dysbiosis. Recent studies show that the imbalance of the microbiota accompanied by a state of hyperpermeability of the intestinal mucosa (Leaky Gut Syndrome) is related to a difficult management of obesity [14] Thus, the use of suitable probiotics would be an important complementary therapy.

The younger an individual, the more intense the mechanism of stress support through food becomes. The use of bupropion associated with topiramate in an intra-gastric balloon protocol has assisted patients in the final periods of balloon use, as well as in the maintenance of weight loss [15].

Drug makers struggle to find viable treatments for this global epidemic. Effective medications to control obesity have proved difficult to develop. The circuits responsible for appetite are outweighed by those who control other important functions, including mood swings, increasing the risk of side effects. The most devastating to the field was the failure of drugs designed to block receptors in the brain that respond to appetite-stimulating chemicals called cannabinoids, where in 2008 the FDA advised doctors not to prescribe them due to the risk of suicidal tendencies.

In patients with morbid obesity, the IGB can be considered a bridge for surgery or a temporary therapeutic treatment in patients not temporary fit into criteria for surgery [16]. Medical therapy should be weighed on a case-by-case basis and integrated into a multidisciplinary approach, such as a diet prescribed by a dietitian with experience in the area and adapted to each patient. A program of appropriate exercises, cognitive therapy, and pharmacological therapy such as sibutramine and orlistat are also implemented.

Association of two drugs is well tolerated and effective in increasing weight loss in obese patients, such as sibutramine and orlistat, drugs with different mechanisms and action [17].

Studies have shown that the results obtained with the implantation of the IGB can be optimized if, in addition to the technique, there is an objective compliance with low-calorie eating plans or the association with sibutramine, thus avoiding some side effects after its removal, like weight recovery after 6 months of treatment.

The goal of obesity treatment is to prevent or mitigate the morbidity associated with being overweight and not just to reach the patient's ideal weight. Pharmacological treatments always combined with diets and physical exercises are indicated for those who have not responded to behavioral approaches.

Orlistat is one of the available antiobesity agents which, acting by inhibiting gastrointestinal lipases, can reduce the absorption of lipids ingested in diet by up to 30%. It remains as an approved drug for long-term treatment of obesity.

Liraglutide is used to treat type 2 diabetes, mimicking an intestinal hormone called *glucagon-like peptide 1* that increases insulin sensitivity and slows down stomach emptying, thus giving a sensation of precocious satiety, like the effect of the IGB, but more pleasant. It is a good choice of drug for use after balloon withdrawal.

In Table 30.3 are given the most commonly used antiobesity drugs that can be used in association with the IGB, when necessary. These may be prescribed during or after the use of the prosthesis.

Weight Regain After Intragastric Balloon Removal

The treatment of weight regain after IGB is done with dietary and physical activity orientation [19]. In cases of excessive regain, depending on the patient's commitment, the use of drugs as a treatment aid is a viable option.

Although the association of antiobesity drugs in patients with weight regain is common practice in endocrinologists' offices, there is little data on the long-term results with this type of approach. Of the antiobesity drugs already mentioned, liraglutide, a GLP-1 receptor agonist (glucagon-like peptide-1), initially launched for the treatment of diabetes at a dose of (1.2–3.0 mg per day), has good results, superior to the placebo group [20].

Table 30.3 Antiobesity drugs that can be used with the intragastric balloon

Drug	Target
Empatic (zonisamide/ bupropion)	Dopamine and noradrenaline reuptake
Liraglutide	Mimics an intestinal hormone called "glucagon-like peptide-1" that increases insulin sensitivity and slows the emptying of the stomach, thus giving a feeling of early satiety
Orlistat	Supports the hypothesis that partial inhibition of fat absorption produces a significant energy deficit, leading to weight loss Considered a useful addition to diet therapy in the primary care setting
Sibutramine	Is effective in the treatment of obesity, both in weight loss and in its maintenance
Symlin (pramlintide/ metreleptin)	Amylin receptor, leptin receptor Analog of amylin, used for the treatment of diabetes. A valuable tool for the treatment of obesity, for the loss of weight loss with a 2x greater durability when associated with the MEV
Tesofensine	Dopamine, noradrenaline, and serotonin reuptake
Velneperit	Neuropeptide Y/peptide YY receptors

Source: Adapted from *Nature* (p. 878, 2010) [18]

Another GLP-1 receptor agonist, exenatide, has already been tested as adjuvant treatment in patients with adjustable gastric band, with good results.

It is important to remember that the feeling of frustration and fear that often affects these patients can trigger compulsion, increased sugar and carbohydrate intake, and worsen the eating pattern, which aggravates the problem [21]. Understanding the causes of weight regain is an important step in treating it.

The follow-up of the patient by an interdisciplinary team (nutritionist, psychologist, physical educator) is essential.

Final Considerations

In treatment with the intragastric balloon, the use of symptomatic medications is suggested within the first 3-5 days, when symptoms of nausea, vomiting and/or abdominal pain may be present.

The use of PPI (proton pump inhibitors) is indicated during the entire permanence of the balloon in the gastric cavity, in order to prevent symptoms and the appearance of lesions of the gastric mucosa, such as gastric erosions or ulcers.

The use of antiobesity drugs concomitant with intragastric balloon therapy appears to be an effective complement to a comprehensive lifestyle intervention to achieve weight reduction and treat obesity-related comorbidities.

Finally, we must emphasize that the most important in the treatment with intragastric balloon is really the change in lifestyle, in patients of any age, using or not associated drugs during or after the use of the balloon. The need to update consensus statements is constant since the scientific evidence on which they are based undergoes increasingly rapid changes, with new therapeutic alternatives arising frequently.

References

1. Ladenheim EE. Liraglutide and obesity: a review of the data so far. Drug Des Devel Ther. 2015;9:1867–75.
2. Almeida N, et al. O balão intragástrico nas formas graves de obesidade. GE J Port Gastrenterol. 2006;13:220–5.
3. Neto MG, et al. Brazilian Intragastric Balloon Consensus Statement (BIBC): practical guidelines based on experience of over 40,000 cases. Surg Obes Relat Dis. 2018;14:151–61.
4. Coutinho WF, Cabral MD. A farmacoterapia da obesidade nos consensos. Arq Bras Endocrinol Metab, São Paulo. 2000;44(1):91–4.
5. Onge E, Miller S, Motycka C. Liraglutide (Saxenda®) as a treatment for obesity. Food Nutr Sci. 2016;7:227–35.
6. Christou GA, Katsiki N, Kiortsis DN. The current role of Liraglutide in the pharmacotherapy of obesity. Curr Vasc Pharmacol. 2016;14(2):201–7.
7. Nissen LP, et al. Intervenções para tratamento da obesidade: revisão sistemática. Rev. Bras. Med. Farm. Comunidade, Florianópolis-SC, Brasil. 2012;7(24):184–90.
8. Paumgartten FJR. Tratamento farmacológico da Obesidade: a perspectiva da saúde pública. Cad Saúde Pública, Rio de Janeiro. 2011;27(3):404–5.
9. Camilleri M. Combining therapies to personalize and optimize treatment. Washington, D.C.: DDW; 2018.
10. Machado ACC, et al. Avaliação da associação da terapêutica medicamentosa e a terapia cognitivo comportamental no tratamento da obesidade. Rev Bras Med. 2002;59(1/2):47–53.
11. Halpern A, Mancini MC. O tratamento da obesidade no paciente portador de hipertensão arterial. Revista Brasileira de Hipertensão. 2000;7(2):166–71.
12. DO Prado CN, et al. Phytotherapic use in the treatment of obesity/O uso de fitoterapicos no tratamento da obesidade. Revista Brasileira de Obesidade, Nutrição e Emagrecimento. 2010;4(19):14. Academic OneFile, Accessed 28 Feb 2018.
13. Verrengia EC, Kinoshita SAT, Amadei JL. Medicamentos Fitoterápicos no Tratamento da Obesidade. UNICIÊNCIAS. 2013;17:53–8.
14. DISBIOSE e Obesidade. Conexões e Curiosidades: Hábitos Saudáveis. Essential Nutrition, ed.10. 2017.
15. Boof RM. Efeito de uma intervenção interdisciplinar baseada no modelo transteórico de mudança de comportamento em adolescentes comsobrepeso ou obesidade. 110f. Tese (Doutorado em Psicologia) – PUCRS: Paraná; 2017.
16. Mazure RA, et al. Adherencia y fidelidad en el paciente tratado con balón intragástrico. Nutr Hosp Madrid. 2014;29(1):50–6.
17. Halpern A, et al. Experiência clínica com o uso conjunto de sibutramina e orlistat em pacientes obesos, vol 44(1). Arq Bras Endocrinol Metab: São Paulo; 2000. p. 103–5.
18. Heidi L. Slim spoils for obesity drugs: drug makers struggle to find viable treatments for global epidemic. Nature. 2010;468:878.
19. Quintas S. Análise de uma amostra de indivíduos após remoção do balão intragástrico e do seu acompanhamento nutricional. Porto: FCNAUP; 2009.
20. Conte SC, De Campos SB. Perspectivas de perda de peso com uso de liraglutida: revisão da literatura. BJSCR. 2014–2015;9(1):84–90.
21. Pajecki D, et al. Tratamento de curto prazo com liraglutide no reganho de peso após cirurgia bariátrica. Rev Col Bras Cir. 2012;40(3):191–5.

Nutritional Follow-Up During Intragastric Balloon Treatment

31

Gabriel Cairo Nunes and Lyz Bezerra Silva

Introduction

Treatment for obesity and overweight is based on an association of medical, nutritional, psychotherapeutic, and exercise-oriented approach. Such therapy necessarily includes a hypocaloric diet (800–1500 Kcal a day), the follow-up of a dietitian with specific experience in the area, and appropriate individual adaptation [1].

After intragastric balloon placement, most patients experience varying degrees of gastrointestinal discomfort, ranging from slight nausea and colic to vomiting, reflux, and dehydration. That is why, at the beginning of treatment, the diet should consist of foods that can easily be cleared by the stomach and then followed by a gradual increase in food consistency in accordance with the individual's degree of tolerance [2].

Diet Progression

The transition from a liquid diet to solids is made in accordance with the patient's adaptation to the balloon and the reduction of the initial symptoms. Ganc et al. [3] recommend that in the first 3 days food intake should be restricted to cold liquids without any lactose, such as gelatin, water, coconut water, fruit popsicles, and sweet lime juice; from the fourth to the eleventh day, any liquid would be permitted, taken in sips and small total amounts and with a caloric value of around 800 Kcal; from the twelfth to the eighteenth day, soft foods can be administered (always respecting the calorie intake restriction);

G. C. Nunes
Department of Endoscopy, University of São Paulo (USP), São Paulo, SP, Brazil

L. B. Silva (✉)
Department of Surgery, Federal University of Pernambuco, Recife, PE, Brazil

© Springer Nature Switzerland AG 2020
M. Galvao Neto et al. (eds.), *Intragastric Balloon for Weight Management*,
https://doi.org/10.1007/978-3-030-27897-7_31

and from then on, the restriction on food texture is decreased and any food can be used within the caloric intake limit of 1000 Kcal a day for as long as the balloon is kept in place.

Preferably, food should be eaten in small amounts several times a day, taking care that the patient chews well and eats slowly. Sallet et al. [4] suggest a liquid diet for the first few days and then an individualized diet with a caloric value of up to 1000 Kcal per day. Similarly, Lopez et al. [5] recommend that on the day after IGB placement, isotonic liquids should be given, progressing gradually in the following days to solid foods but never more than 1000 Kcal a day.

In line with other authors, Kotzampassi et al. [6] state that in the first 3 days, the patient must remain on a liquid diet gradually evolving to consume semisolids and solids.

In addition to recommending a liquid diet for 3 days, Dastis et al. [7] encourage the consumption of protein-rich beverages. After this initial period, the dietary progression should be adapted to the patient with a limit of 1000 Kcal per day, consisting of 15% proteins, 30% or less of lipids, and 55% of carbohydrates. Also, in their view, the consumption of alcohol must be strictly avoided. De Castro et al. [8] consider that the patient should be on a liquid diet and gradually transition to a solid diet with a maximum daily calorie intake of 1000 Kcal. They differ from other authors, however, as they recommend the use of a vitamin complex. Gottig et al. [9] favor a liquid diet for the first 3 weeks and a gradual introduction of solid foods in the fourth week, whereas Gumurdulu et al. [10] recommend a liquid diet up till the end of the first week and then gradual individualized diet adjustment with a calorie intake maximum of 1100 Kcal a day.

As shown, there is agreement in the literature regarding the calorie intake (around 1000 Kcal) and the need for a gradual evolution from the initial liquid diet to normal textures of food. In our experience, it is essential that the dietary progression is individualized, thereby reducing the patients' complaints regarding the food and nutritional impacts in that early stage of greatest gastric stasis [2]. It must also be remembered that a large percentage of obese patients take oral antidiabetic agents, in which case it is advisable to monitor glycemia and avoid any risk of hypoglycemia [11].

At all stages, patients are advised to avoid any food containing sucrose, not just for weight loss considerations but also to protect the balloon, given the occurrence of gastric stasis due to proton pump inhibitors' use and the presence of the prosthesis itself—conditions that facilitate the proliferation of fungi on the IGB surface. They must also strictly avoid consuming any alcohol or carbonated drinks, albeit there is still some controversy regarding their effects. They may be related to the liberation of gastric acids in the case of alcohol, and both alcohol and soda may lead to the relaxation of the inferior sphincter, fostering gastric emptying, an effect precisely the opposite of the mechanism the implantation of the IGB is intended to achieve. Another valuable practice is to have the patient register the daily nutritional intake by keeping a diary [2, 11].

Table 31.1 comprises an outline of how the dietary progression can be achieved:

Table 31.1 Outline of how to achieve the dietary progression

Stages	Average number of days	Average calorie intake	Examples of suitable food	Average volume/time
1. Liquid	3 days	500	Weak teas, isotonic sports drinks, coconut water, light strained soups, jellies, fruit popsicles	30–50 mL/20/30 minutes
2. Completely liquid	4 days	700	Yoghurts, skimmed milk, fruit milk shakes, fruit juices	100–150 mL/hour
3. Puree/liquefied creams	7 days	700	Purees, softened fruits, porridge, fruit milk shakes	4–5 meals a day; 100–150 g per meal
4. Soft food	7 days	750	Softened vegetables, ground meats, cheeses	5–6 meals a day; 200 g each meal
5. General/normal texture	3 weeks after implantation	800–1000	Varied and individually adapted	4–6 meals a day
6. Completely liquid	3 days prior to removal	750	Weak teas, isotonic sports drinks, coconut water, light broths, jellies, fruit popsicles	6–7 meals a day; 200 mL each meal

- *Stage 1*: This initial stage begins with cold liquid foods and lasts for roughly 3 days, which is the period when patients are most liable to complain of vomiting, gastric reflux, and a feeling of gastric satiety. The recommended foods are isotonic drinks, coconut water, water, natural fruit juice popsicles, natural fruit juice diluted with water, frozen isotonic drinks, or frozen coconut water and protein supplement beverages.

  The volume of the daily food intake is also very important given the contraction effort the stomach makes in an endeavor to expel the balloon. The dietary volume usually tolerated is in the range of 30–50 mL every 20/30 minutes provided that the patient is following his or her normal daily routine and taking 10-minute walks, three times a day. During this stage, it is important to pay careful attention to any clinical signs, because in some cases, the gastric discomfort is so frequent that dehydration may occur to a variable extent and may lead to the need for intravenous hydration. It must also be borne in mind that patients using hypoglycemiants as part of their overweight treatment must stop using the medication during the first week when the diet, albeit rich in simple carbohydrates, provides a calorie intake of less than 500 Kcal a day.

- *Stage 2*: After the third day, the diet enters stage two. During this stage, the symptoms of gastric distress tend to become less intense and the volume intake the patient can tolerate increases. The kind of foods included during this stage are strained soups with no added oils, diet or light jellies, clear teas (chamomile, lemon balm, and apple), natural fruit juices diluted with water, skimmed milk, light and skimmed milk yogurts, and protein supplement drinks.

The recommended volumes are 100 to 150 mL every hour. That may be varied according to the degree of gastric discomfort experienced after ingestion. On average, this stage lasts for 4 days.

- *Stage 3*: This stage begins after the first week has elapsed and the diet evolves to include food in the form of creams or pastes. The foods usually offered are creamed soups, vegetable purees, curds, fruit milk shakes, and porridges using skimmed milk.
- *Stage 4*: Two weeks after IGB implantation, stage four begins and a light diet is introduced. Diet intake is regulated to five or six meals a day with limited calorie content. The volume of each meal is around 200 mL or roughly five spoons. Foods in this stage are soft either through cooking or going through a food processor or blender. The total calorie intake varies from 800 to 1000 Kcal a day and consists of soft or cooked fruits (e.g., banana, papaya, grated apple, and cantaloupe), light yogurts or skimmed milk yogurts with added vitamins, cottage-type cheese, natural juices, cooked or braised greens or vegetables, minced, shredded, or pre-ground meats, and whole wheat bread.
- *Stage 5*: After the third week, normal-textured food is introduced. At this stage, the recommendation is that the diet should be low calorie and every effort should be made to foster and encourage healthy eating habits. During stage five, the diet should be administered in the form of five or six meals a day with a total daily calorie intake not exceeding 1000 Kcal. To help with diet control, it is helpful if the patient keeps a food intake diary that can be shown to the nutrition team at the monthly follow-up sessions [2, 11].

Adjustable Intragastric Balloon

The adjustable IGB makes it possible to increase the balloon volume and achieve extra weight loss. The idea underlying volumetric progression is that when the balloon volume is increased, it will make gastric emptying increasingly difficult thereby diminishing food ingestion. After an adjustment of the balloon, the patient should go back to the diet protocol used at the beginning when the prosthesis was newly implanted but this time, the evolution to a more normal-textured type of food will be faster.

- Stage 1: Restricted liquid diet (800 Kcal) for 2 days + 12 hours total fasting prior to readjustment.
- Stage 2: Completely liquid diet (700 Kcal) for 1–2 days after the adjustment.
- Stage 3: Liquefied cream or paste (700 Kcal) for 2–4 days.
- Stage 4: Foods softened by cooking or braising (759 Kcal) for 2–4 days.
- Stage 5: Low-calorie food of normal texture (800/1000 Kcal) up until a new IGB adjustment or removal of the balloon.

Volumetric Reduction of the Adjustable IGB Due to Patient Discomfort

Most patients experience some degree of discomfort (nausea, belching, heartburn, reflux, vomiting, and colic), and those conditions can get worse if there is no suitable dietary control. In some cases, the symptoms are so strong that it is chosen to reduce the volume of the IGB to facilitate gastric emptying. Ideally, any reduction in the IGB volume would only be done when the patient was correctly adhering to the planned diet but even so was experiencing considerable difficulty to adapt. However, in those cases, where there has been a transgression of the diet, then the option should be to go back to a stage one (liquid) diet for 2 days and then reassess the symptoms and restart the dietary progression process until the normal-textured food stage (stage five) is reached.

We have observed that some studies report that balloon volume reduction does indeed relieve the symptoms referred to above, but that there is an accompanying gain in weight or at least a stabilization of the weight loss process in that period. For that reason, before deciding to reduce the volume of the balloon, it is better to try some dietary modifications first.

Intolerance and Food Impaction

One of the IGB's two main functions is to delay gastric emptying causing an increased feeling of satiety. The intensity of the food impaction needs to be adjusted individually for each patient. Individuals vary greatly in their degree of tolerance of dietetic volume. That being so, the use of an alimentary diary can be very useful to identify intolerance and make the necessary adjustments to the diet.

The presence of gastric food residues is a frequent condition causing foul-smelling belching due to the putrefaction of the food, heartburn due to excess production of acid (even with the use of proton pump inhibitors), reflux, and, in some cases, spontaneous vomiting and gastric colic. The most efficient tool for identifying gastric emptying after a meal is the alimentary diary in which the patient's feelings after ingesting food are registered, thereby making it feasible to readjust the volume and distribution of the alimentation. It should be noted that proteins of animal origin, including red meat, are the type of food most commonly associated to belching, colic, and reflux. The connection of those foods to the aforementioned symptoms is only to be expected because they are linked to a greater liberation of satiety inducing hormones, which, in a cascade effect, reduces gastric emptying and intestinal motility, leading to an increased feeling of satiety [12, 13].

When there are symptoms associated to food stasis, it is recommended to revert to a stage two diet for at least 3 days so that the food residues present in the gastric cavity can be cleared. It is well known that, depending on their macronutrient composition, liquids are capable of fostering gastric emptying, resulting in a reduced feeling of satiety and possibly resulting in a greater energetic ingestion [14–16].

Protein Content of the Diet

Altering the macronutrient composition can possibly bring changes in weight loss patterns. However, restriction on energetic nutrients is the main independent factor determining weight loss [17, 18]. Protein-rich diets offer a high level of energy spending compared to carbohydrates or lipids, due to the high thermogenic capacity of such nutrients with a consequent loss in weight [12, 13].

The thermic effect of food (TEF) is the energy spent in ingesting, digesting, absorbing, using, and storing the ingested nutrients. It represents from 5% to 15% of the total energy spent, which shows how important it is in regulating body weight and the energy equilibrium. In the case of a balanced diet, this effect can represent an energy spending of 10–15% of the diet's calorie content but when macronutrients are ingested separately, the proteins, carbohydrates, and lipids present thermic effects of 20–30%, 5–10%, and 0–3%, respectively, of the total of ingested calories. The thermic effect occurs in two distinct stages: the cephalic or facultative stage occurs through the action of the sympathetic nervous system activated by the sensorial aspects of the diet; the gastrointestinal or obligatory stage is characterized by the energy spent in the process of absorption and usage of the nutrients in terms of the consumption of ATP [19, 20]. The diet's caloric content and composition are among the most important factors modulating the TEF [20–22].

Protein is the most thermogenic nutrient and leads to an energy spending of 19% of the energy ingested simply for its utilization and storage, whereas lipids only require 3% for the same metabolic feats [23–25]. At the same time, the thermal effect of proteins is 50–100% higher than that of carbohydrates and that is generally attributed to the high metabolic costs of forging peptide links, ureagenesis, and gluconeogenesis [26]. Protein is also associated to controlling the appetite because of a more prolonged satiety due to the fact that it stimulates the secretion of certain satiety-inducing hormones such as cholecystokinin (cck), glucagon-like-peptide 1 (GLP-1), and peptide-YY (PYY) [25–27]. That is why the general stage of diet should involve an average 30% of foods that are a source of proteins.

In prescription of diets, we use many dairy-based foods such as skimmed milk, light yoghurt, and bland cheese. That is a way to enhance the consumption of calcium stemming from a regular diet and also the protein content. Some studies have shown that dairy foods rich in calcium seem to favor the loss of body fat [28, 29], while others suggest that it favors the maintenance of the fat loss achieved through the weight loss process [30, 31]. Several studies have identified a direct association between calcium ingestion and body fat loss [32, 33]. The mechanisms reducing fatty tissue associated to the ingestion of calcium in the diet are now much clearer. One hypothesis is that the formation of calcium salts in the digestive tract facilitates the loss of fat via the feces [34].

Diet for IGB Removal

The IGB causes a reduction in the velocity of gastric emptying, which means that in order for the stomach to be completely "clean" for adequate removal of the balloon, it is necessary to administer a totally liquid diet for at least 3 days prior to the procedure and, in addition, impose a total fast of 8 hours (stage six). Some authors like Kotzampassi et al. [6] have reported the use of sodas and fizzy beverages to facilitate gastric emptying, but there are no reports confirming as to whether that practice brings in better or worse results than a liquid diet and a period of fasting.

Follow-Up After Removal

In groups that treat patients who have undergone bariatric surgery, the rate of adherence to the nutritional consultations is low [35–37]. The same phenomenon is common among patients who make use of IGBs, as we have observed that 50% come back for follow-up fewer than six times in a year. In our practice, specifically, the figure is 47.2% [2]. That evasion of the scheduled consultations can have a negative impact on long-term results. The data attesting that fact can readily be found in the body of literature addressing weight loss treatments [38–40].

References

1. Herron DM. The surgical management of severe obesity. Mount Sinai J Med. 2004;71:63–71.
2. Nunes GC, Pajecki D, de Melo ME, Mancini MC, de Cleva R, Santo MA. Assessment of weight loss with the intragastric balloon in patients with different degrees of obesity. Surg Laparosc Endosc Percutan Tech. 2017;27:e83–6.
3. Ganc A, Ganc RL, De Paula A. A prospective evaluation of a new intra-gastric balloon for the treatment of obesity; a two center experience. In: DDW 15–20 May 2004, New Orleans, 2004.
4. Sallet JA. Balão intragástrico: gastroplastia endoscópica para o tratamento da obesidade. São Paulo: Caminho Editorial; 2001. p. 19–31.
5. Lopez-Nava G, et al. BioEnterics® intragastric balloon (BIB®). Single ambulatory center Spanish experience with 714 consecutive patients treated with one or two consecutive balloons. Obes Surg. 2011;21(1):5–9.
6. Kotzampassi K, et al. 500 Intragastric balloons: what happens 5 years thereafter? Obes Surg. 2012;22(6):896–903.
7. Dastis NS, et al. Intragastric balloon for weight loss: results in 100 individuals followed for at least 2.5 years. Endoscopy. 2009;41(7):575–80.
8. De Castro ML, et al. Safety and effectiveness of gastric balloons associated with hypocaloric diet for the treatment of obesity. Revista española de enfermedades digestivas. 2013;105(9):529–36.
9. Göttig S, et al. Analysis of safety and efficacy of intragastric balloon in extremely obese patients. Obes Surg. 2009;19(6):677–83.
10. Gümürdülü Y, et al. Long-term effectiveness of BioEntericsintragastric balloon in obese patients. Turk J Gastroenterol. 2013;24(5):387–91.
11. Nunes GC, de Vasconcellos IF. O balão que emagrece. 1st ed. São Paulo: Livrus; 2014.

12. Anderson GH, Tecimer SN, Shah D, Zafar TA. Protein source, quantity and time of consumption determine the effect of proteins on short-term food intake in young men. J Nutr. 2004;134(11):3011–5.
13. Paddon-Jones D, Westman E, Matter RD, Wolfe RR, Astrup A, Westerterp-Plantenga M. Protein, weight management, and satiety. Am J Clin Nut. 2008;87(5):1558S–61S.
14. Haber GB, Heaton KW, Murphy D, Burroughs LF. Depletion and disruption of dietary fiber. Effects on satiety, plasma-glucose, and serum- insulin. Lancet. 1977;2:679–82.
15. Zijlstra N, Mars M, Wijk RA, Westerterp-Plantenga MS, Holst JJ, Graaf C. Effect of viscosity on appetite and gastro-intestinal hormones. Physiol Behav. 2009;97(1):68–75.
16. Martens JI, Westerterp-Platenga MS. Mode of consumption plays a role in alleviating hunger and thirst. Obesity. 2012;20(3):517–24.
17. Heymsfield SB, Van Mierlo CAJ, Van Der Knaap HCM, Heo M, Frier HI. Weight management using a meal replacement strategy: meta and pooling analysis from six studies. Int J Obes. 2003;27(5):537–49.
18. Almeida JC, Rodrigues TC, Silva FM, Azevedo MJ. Revisão sistemática de dietas de emagrecimento: papel dos componentes dietéticos. Arq Bras Endocrinol Metab. 2009;59(5):673–87.
19. Tappy L. Thermic effect of food and sympathetic nervous system activity in humans. Reprod Nutr Dev. 1996;36:391–7.
20. Hermsdorff HHM, Monteiro JBR, Mourão DM, Leite MCT. Termogênese induzida pela dieta: uma revisão sobre seu papel no balanço energético e no controle de peso. Rev Bras Nutr Clin. 2003;18(1):37–41.
21. Jonge L, Bray GA. The thermic effect of food and obesity: a critical review. Obes Res. 1997;5(6):622–31.
22. Labayen I, Martínez JA. Distribución de macronutrientes de la dieta y regulación del peso y composición corporal: papel de la ingesta lipídica en la obesidad. An Sist Sanit Navar. 2002;25(Suppl.1):79–90.
23. Crovetti R, Porrini M, Santangelo A, Testolin G. The influence of thermic effect of food on satiety. Eur J Clin Nutr. 1998;52(7):482–8.
24. Westerterp-Plantenga MS, Rolland V, Wilson SAJ, Westerterp KR. Satiety related to 24 h diet-induced thermogenesis during high protein/carbohydrate vs high fat diets measured in a respiration chamber. Eur J Clin Nutr. 1999;53(6):495–502.
25. Doucet E, Tremblay A. Food intake, energy balance and body weight control. Eur J Clin Nutr. 1997;51(12):849–55.
26. Johnston CS, Day CS, Swan PD. Postprandial thermogenesis is increased 100% on a high-protein, low-fat diet versus a high carbohydrate, low-fat diet in healthy, young women. J Am Coll Nutr. 2002;21(1):55–61.
27. Astrup A, Raben A, Geiker N. The role of higher protein diets in weight control and obesity-related comorbidities. Int J Obes. 2014;39:721–6.
28. Haraguchi FK, de Abreu WC, de Paula H. Proteínas do soro do leite: composição, propriedades nutricionais, aplicações no esporte e benefícios para a saúde humana. Rev Nutr [online]. 2006;19(4):479–88. https://doi.org/10.1590/S1415-52732006000400007. ISSN 16789865
29. Westerterp-Plantenga MS. The significance of protein in food intake and body weight regulation. Curr Opin Clin Nutr Metab Care. 2003;6:635–8.
30. Pereira MA, Jacobs DR Jr, Horm L, Slaterry ML, Kartashov AI, Ludwing DS. Dairy consumption, obesity, and the insulin resistance syndrome in young adults: the CARDIA study. JAMA. 2002;287(16):2081–9.
31. Zemel MB, Thompson W, Milstead A, Morris K, Campbell P. Calcium and dairy acceleration of weight and fat loss during energy restriction in obese adults. Obes Res. 2004;12(4):582–90.
32. Zemel MB, Richards J, Mathis S, Milstead A, Gebhardt L, Silva E. Dairy augmentation of total and central fat loss in obese subjects. Int J Obes. 2005;29(4):391–7.
33. Fiorito LM, Ventura AK, Mitchell DG, Smiciklas-Wright H, Birch LL. Girls' dairy intake, energy intake, and weight status. J Am Diet Assoc. 2006;106:1851–5.
34. Estever EA, Paulino EJ, Rodrigues CAA. Ingestão dietética de cálcio e adiposidade em mulheres adultas. Rev Nutr Campinas. 2010;23(4):543–52.

35. Shen R, Dugay G, Rajaram K, Cabrera I, Siegel N, Ren CJ. Impact of patient follow-up on weight loss after bariatric surgery. Obes Surg. 2004;14(4):514–9. https://doi.org/10.1381/096089204323013523.
36. Harper J, Madan AK, Ternovits GA, Tichansky DS. What happens to patients who do not follow-up after bariatric surgery? Am Surg. 2007;73(2):181–4.
37. Lanyon RI, Maxwell BM, Kraft AJ. Prediction of long-term outcome after gastric bypass surgery. Obes Surg. 2009;19(4):439–45. https://doi.org/10.1007/11695-008-9740-3.
38. Pi-Sunyer X, Astrup A, Fujioka K, et al. SCALE Obesity and Prediabetes NN8022-1839 Study Group. A randomized, controlled trial of 3.0 mg of Liraglutide in weight management. N Engl J Med. 2015;373:11–22.
39. James WP, Astrup A, Finer N, et al. Effect of sibutramine on weight maintenance after wenausea, weight loss: a randomised trial. STORM Study Group Sibutramine trial of obesity reduction and maintenance. Lancet. 2000;356:2119–25.
40. Switzer NJ, Merani S, Sklubeni D, et al. Quality of follow-up: systematic review of the research in bariatric surgery. Ann Surg. 2016;263:875–80.

Psychotherapy in Intragastric Balloon Treatment

32

Hélio Tonelli and Uliana Fernanda Pozzobon

Introduction

Over the past few decades, obesity has been considered a major public health problem since, only in the United States, an estimated two-thirds of the adult population and 30% of children and adolescents are overweight or obese [1]. The BioEnterics intragastric balloon (BIB) is considered a nonsurgical and nonpharmacological, reversible, and repeatable treatment [3], widely used for weight reduction in obese patients who have had unsatisfactory results in clinical and multidisciplinary treatment of obesity [2], as well as for minimizing surgical risks in the preoperative preparation of bariatric surgery in morbidly obese patients [3]. Several studies have shown its efficacy and safety, remarkably in short-term treatments, particularly when associated with a multidisciplinary follow-up. Fernandes et al. (2012) systematically reviewed nine randomized trials involving 395 BIB users, concluding that the procedure is secure, but without evidence showing its superiority when compared to the traditional obesity management. However, these authors highlighted that the included studies were very heterogeneous both clinically and methodologically, emphasizing that factors associated with both weight loss and its maintenance were motivation and encouragement to change habits. Considering that, in addition to weight loss, the main goal of obesity treatment is to maintain weight at desirable levels, few studies have evaluated the efficacy of long-term BIB treatment. Kotzampassi et al. [4] followed patients for 5 years after BIB removal, showing that the efficacy for weight loss and its long-term maintenance is a direct function of acceptance and adherence to

H. Tonelli (✉)
Department of Psychiatry, Caetano Marchesini Clinic and FAE Business School, Curitiba, PR, Brazil

U. F. Pozzobon
Psychology, Curitiba, PR, Brazil

© Springer Nature Switzerland AG 2020
M. Galvao Neto et al. (eds.), *Intragastric Balloon for Weight Management*,
https://doi.org/10.1007/978-3-030-27897-7_32

multidisciplinary management from the beginning of the treatment, what is in full accordance with the main guidelines for the treatment of obesity, which advise therapeutic strategies combining changes in lifestyle habits, physical exercises, and behavioral treatment [5], routinely prescribed and supervised by a multiprofessional team.

Nevertheless, mental health consultants attending patients on BIB treatment should not act only within the period of 6 months in which patients usually remain with the balloon, but also after its removal, when they are under greater risk of obesity recurrence. The behavioral treatment of obesity, which can be done using different psychotherapeutic techniques, is mainly aimed at providing a mental structure that allows one to reach the goals of the treatment, that is, losing weight and/or controlling dysfunctional eating behaviors, and does not necessarily treat the problem of obesity directly. Indeed, obesity has been increasingly considered a medical condition in which behavior is only a variable out of a multifactorial etiologic complex [7], which, for instance, involves low-level brain inflammatory processes [8, 9], brain insulin resistance [11], and brain influences of intestinal microbiome changes [8, 10] secondary to obesity, all of them known to be associated with behaviors that facilitate weight gain. Hence, for a considerable proportion of patients with obesity, psychological issues are not primarily etiological [7], but are consequences of multiple pathological processes disrupting brain neurotransmitter circuits underlying the processing of rewards, mood, eating behavior, and cognitive control. Consequently, some cognitive, emotional, and behavioral changes commonly observed while some individuals are obese might be reversed following weight loss. On the other hand, many psychiatric disorders apparently increase the risk of obesity, either because they increase the odds of dysfunctional eating behaviors and/or a sedentary lifestyle, or because of the chronic use of obesogenic drugs for their treatment [12], reasons why obese patients with comorbid psychiatric disorders must be properly evaluated before receiving pharmacological, surgical or psychotherapeutic treatments for obesity.

Psychotherapeutic Approaches to Obesity

Although there are no studies comparing the efficacy of different psychotherapeutic approaches in patients under treatment with the intragastric balloon, cognitive-behavioral psychotherapy (CBT) has been the most studied technique. For instance, Majanovik et al. [14] compared the efficacy of BIB and CBT for weight reduction and its effects on metabolic variables during 6 months. Participants treated with BIB significantly lost more weight and showed more improvements in several metabolic parameters when compared to those receiving CBT; therefore, the combination of BIB with CBT may favor even more consistent improvements. On the other hand, Takihata et al. [15] failed to demonstrate superiority of BIB treatment when compared to an intensive lifestyle modification program for weight loss in Japanese super-obese participants.

To date, the same guidelines used for the psychotherapeutic approach to obesity guide the psychological treatment of patients on BIB treatment (and, somehow, the same occurs with the psychotherapy of bariatric patients, a topic that has not yet been satisfactorily studied).

First, it is important to keep in mind that *cognitive-behavioral techniques* should be differentiated from *interventions to change habits or lifestyles*, although there is not always a clear distinction between them [6]. Habits/lifestyle change interventions comprise actions to stimulate dietary changes and physical activity [6], which may use behavioral techniques such as self-monitoring, goal setting, stimulus control, problem solving, and relapse prevention [5, 6, 13]. Cognitive-behavioral techniques of CBT, in turn, use such strategies associated with a *cognitive* component of the therapy aiming at cognitive restructuring [5, 6], through the evaluation and modification of thoughts, beliefs, emotions, self-attributions, self-esteem, and self-efficacy related to weight loss [13]. The terminological inaccuracy of psychotherapeutic interventions for weight loss tends to complicate the study of the efficacy of the techniques allegedly used, since they are poorly defined not only as to their nature (i.e., counseling, coaching, or psychotherapy), but also as to who conducts the treatment (psychologist, psychiatrist, nutritionist, physical educator, etc.) [7].

Self-Monitoring

Patients on BIB should be encouraged to observe and take note of their attitudes and behaviors regarding food, physical activity, and their weight. Self-monitoring is considered one of the pillars of behavioral treatment of obesity [17]. Systematic recordings of diet, weight, and exercise seem to increase the awareness of behaviors leading to weight gain [18], predicting weight maintenance after bariatric surgery, along with the ability to control eating impulses [16]. This is because individuals who are accustomed to and well trained in self-monitoring can reinforce healthy behaviors by better observing their progress [18].

In a systematic review of the literature, Burke et al. [18] conclude that the higher frequency of self-monitoring is consistently and significantly associated with greater weight loss, although these authors were not able to determine the exact frequency that made the difference. These authors add that increasing the use of technology to aid in self-monitoring, facilitating it, may increase adherence to this strategy and their findings suggest that being male, having better social support, lower body mass index (BMI) and belonging to a structured weight loss program are indicators of more efficient self-monitoring.

Peterson et al. [17] studied the impact of three components of food self-monitoring (frequency, consistency and comprehension) on weight and concluded that frequent and consistent records (i.e., records maintained overtime on a homogeneous basis) are more efficient for the maintenance of weight changes, as well as that comprehension (the detailing with which the records were made) did not add any benefit to the treatment.

Goal Setting

BIB users benefit from learning behavioral strategies that help them achieve what they want in terms of weight loss. One of these strategies is to set clear and tangible goals. The process of setting goals, done by a patient assisted by her/his therapist, in addition to reinforcing the therapeutic alliance, is acknowledged as an evidence-based behavioral change strategy, for it is specific, measurable, and palpable [21]. Well-established goals influence individual performance by directing attention and effort, minimizing the effect of distractors, and increasing energy, motivation and persistence for them to be achieved [19]. This strategy, therefore, has a real moderating effect on cognition, favoring a highly attentive state of mind, in which competitive thoughts and feelings are more easily overcome [20]. Such a state of mind would override habitual executive processes, interfering in unconscious psychological automatisms related to food and reinforced by habit, modifying food perception and motivation for eating.

Motivation for the pursuit of previously established goals is also enhanced when they are properly defined. Moreover, goals (or mental representations of desired outcomes) incorporate a fundamental aspect of mental functioning, the reward-mediated learning, in that, when goals are achieved, the patient is rewarded, what reinforces the behavior leading to the achievement of her or his goals. Hence, clearly stated goals eliminate ambiguities and favor mental performance for them to be achieved through cognitive mechanisms of increasing attention to them.

Stimulus Control

Eating behavior in obese people is influenced by a phenomenon called *cue-potentiated eating* [22] or *unplanned eating*, characterized by a much more intense behavior of searching for food after an exposure to whichever food cue. Initially meaningless stimuli may acquire new cognitive, affective, and motivational roles when they occur in certain contexts favoring the association between internal (e.g., hunger) and external events (e.g., the pleasant odor of the food, or even a restaurant logo).

Food cues are important in regulating homeostasis because, by learning what they predict, animals can anticipate their needs rather than simply react to them [27]. Food cues can influence the release of intestinal peptides and activate mental representations of foods that include their sensory details – for instance, taste and texture – as well as their affective and motivational properties, which together determine their "desirability" [26]. Thus, food cues can trigger cravings in the same way as some drugs do [23, 36], even in moments of satiety, leading to unplanned eating. This is because food cues acquire the ability to activate central reward systems in a similar way to food [24], and such activation may be amplified in brains of obese individuals, who additionally have less activity within circuits processing cognitive control [25].

Stimulus control interventions aim to improve pathological eating behaviors by identifying and modifying environmental factors that trigger them [28]. However, such interventions can be a major challenge in modern Western societies characterized by environments where food cues are abundant. Additionally, two other points make this approach even more challenging: first, functional neuroimaging studies show that in obesity there is a decrease of the activity of brain structures associated with cognitive control, such as the dorsolateral prefrontal cortex, after the exposure to food cues [25]; second, there are individual, temperamental, differences in the ability of cognitively controlling eating behaviors [29, 30].

Problem-Solving

Problem-solving is a cognitive-behavioral technique used in different medical and psychological contexts, aimed at assisting the development of adaptive solutions to everyday problems and strengthening adherence to medical treatments [31]. Many patients using BIB will not adhere to diets, physical activity programs, and even multidisciplinary follow-up because they believe the balloon will "do all the hard work," unless they are properly taught about their role in weight loss and its maintenance. Frequently, mistaken expectations about the treatment with an intragastric balloon are even shared by the patients' relatives. Therefore, low adherence to the treatment of obesity usually occurs due to false beliefs and attitudes regarding the role of BIB, lack of motivation and skills, and/or social support to carry out the changes of lifestyles and habits necessary for a consistent weight loss [31].

Structured problem solving techniques can help improving a wide range of medical conditions, including obesity. They comprise, in essence, a process of supervised learning of a method for identifying personal problems underlying specific symptoms leading to weight gain, as well as for developing suitable skills to solve these problems [32, 33]. Individuals suffering from obesity may be encouraged to identify automatic thoughts and affects that trigger dysfunctional eating behaviors (e.g., emotional eating or loss of control of eating) and to discover strategies for their eradication. The technique encompasses different phases, beginning with the delimitation of the problem, its clarification and the elaboration of a plan to approach it, being complemented by a clear establishment of objectives, besides the encouragement to the description of available proposals aiming at the resolution of the problem [32, 33]. It is common for patients treating obesity to have very vague, unreal or hard to solve problems, as well as poorly defined or intangible strategies to deal with these problems. These patients often benefit from the assisted clarification of their goals and the means to achieve them.

Relapse Prevention

Although controversial, the similarity of some eating behaviors in obesity with substance and behavioral dependencies from the phenomenological point of view seems frequently inevitable. The similarity between such phenomena is supported by a series of neuroscientific findings showing superposition of neural pathways in both conditions [23, 36].

Preliminary findings of studies on eating addiction (also known as food addiction) suggest that at least some clinical elements of substance and behavioral additions are present in patients with obesity. They include:

1. Engaging in eating in order to seek effects such as pleasure, euphoria, excitement, or relief from unpleasure.
2. Concern with such behaviors associated to multiple efforts to stop or avoid them.
3. Salience (when a substance or a behavior takes on the meaning of what is most important in the subject's life).
4. Loss of control and
5. Negative consequences of that behavior on the individual's life [34].

Thus, just as it occurs with addicts, individuals suffering from obesity need assistance in order to avoid relapses and to learn to deal with such losses of control. In this sense, it is essential to add that diets stimulate a predominantly cognitive control over food, which is easily lost when one has to deal with a negative affect or an environmental stressor, leading to the abandonment of diets, when not to eating disorders [35], whose risk is already increased in obesity.

Weeks to months before a pathological eating behavior returns in an individual on a diet, dysfunctional emotions and cognitions may already sign that a relapse is on the way. Teaching patients to recognize and develop skills to deal with these unfavorable mental states is the primary goal of relapse prevention. Melemis [37] proposes that relapses of substance disorders involve emotional, mental and physical phases. We believe that they also affect patients receiving treatment for obesity, who may consequently benefit from the relapse prevention approach.

In the emotional phase, patients are not aware of negative emotions favoring relapses and may be more socially isolated, avoiding focusing on their own problems as they pay more attention to the others'. At this stage, there is massive use of rationalizations and therapists can help patients focus on unconscious feelings by increasing attention to four domains of emotional and motivational life which, when neglected, contribute to increased risk of food relapse, and which can be remembered by the acronym HALT (hungry, angry, lonely and tired) [37].

Signs of mental (cognitive) relapses include cravings and thoughts about places, people, and things associated with past uses – consequences of eating behaviors potentiated by food cues –, as well as minimization of the consequences of a relapse, the pursuit of relapse opportunities, and its planning.

Physical relapse occurs when the patient has already engaged in dysfunctional eating, with varying levels of lack of control. Loss of control over eating has been identified not only in major eating disorders, such as bulimia nervosa and binge eating disorder, but also in conditions such as *grazing*, *nibbling*, or *snack eating*, which could be understood as subsyndromal eating disorders [38], where small amounts of food are recurrently consumed without planning between meals.

It is important to keep in mind that many dietary programs endorse several meals per day or small low carb snacks between meals, and that such orientations might be subverted as subsyndromal eating disorders by some obese patients. Therefore, relapse prevention programs should take into account all the complexity of the addicted mind as well as the various clinical facets with which behavioral disorders present themselves.

Cognitive Restructuring

CBT of obesity employs all the techniques discussed above associated with a cognitive component, which encompasses the evaluation and modification of thoughts, beliefs, emotions, and motivations regarding weight loss. Beliefs, the primary therapeutic target of CBT, can be defined as probabilities that a proposition about the world is true [39]. They are mental representations of expectations about the world and things, have a predictive role, and need to be updated so that their predictive and representational roles are increased [39]. Therefore, the role of the CBT therapist in the treatment of obesity is to help patients update deeply rooted dysfunctional beliefs about eating and about their abilities to control eating impulses and lose weight. Dysfunctional beliefs like *being thin is not for me*, *I do not deserve to be thin* or *I will never be able to adhere to a physical exercise routine* consolidate throughout a history of multiple attempts and failures in previous weight loss programs and can endanger the treatment with BIB. They need to be properly evaluated and corrected (updated). In this process of evaluating and correcting false beliefs, the patient should be taught to monitor her or his dysfunctional and automatic thoughts, apply corrections, create healthier alternative responses to them, value minor achievements, and react differently to any weight gain; hence, increasing their self-efficacy [13]. Failures in previous treatments may favor erroneous beliefs about the intragastric balloon, such as the idealization of a treatment that does not require any effort or sacrifice on the part of the patient, which usually results in failure to achieve the expected goals.

Interpersonal Psychotherapy for Obesity

Many patients report that their eating behavior is strongly associated with feelings of pleasure, excitement, and happiness, as well as with relief from displeasure, anhedonia, or unhappiness, reflecting a peculiar relationship between eating and emotion/affectivity, which is highlighted within interpersonal contexts. Contemporary psychology proposes that happiness be composed of three domains: pleasure (*hedonia*), well-being (*eudaimonia*), and interpersonal attachment (*engagement*) [40]. Indeed, it is not uncommon for patients to complain that feelings of loneliness, isolation, and not-belonging guide many of their pathological eating behaviors, notwithstanding that obese individuals have been ostensibly rejected throughout their lives, which is behind strong feelings of social exclusion.

Interpersonal psychotherapy (IPT) is a therapeutic modality that has been shown to be effective in several psychological disorders, whose mechanisms focus on interpersonal processes and aim at increasing social support, reducing interpersonal stress, facilitating emotional processing in social contexts, and increasing of social skills [41]. Group IPT is comparable in efficacy to group CBT in the treatment of overweight patients with Binge Eating Disorder [43]. Recent studies have shown the efficacy of IPT in preventing weight gain in adolescents with high risk for obesity in adulthood [42] and the family-focused interpersonal approach in overweight or obese pre-adolescents with loss of control over eating, particularly in reducing the psychological distress of those children, with a positive impact on their eating behavior [44]. Although there are no studies on the efficacy of IPT in patients being treated with BIB, it is very likely that this technique may particularly benefit patients with eating behaviors triggered by loss of control.

Mindfulness

Therapeutic techniques based on transcendental meditation have been increasingly employed for the treatment of various medical and psychological conditions. Automatic and unconscious thoughts, emotions, and motivations often lie behind intrusive ruminations about the future, the past, and other people [45], leading to dysfunctional psychological and behavioral styles. Mindfulness meditation addresses these mental states through the cultivation of a nonjudgmental psychological state centered in the present, in which every thought, feeling, or sensation that arises in consciousness must be accepted as it actually is [46].

Some encouraged attitudes in mindfulness meditation include an impartial witnessing stance of one's own experiences, avoiding thoughtless conclusions and not falling into the temptation of trying to anticipate things, being open to new possibilities and accepting how things are here and now. Such a stance involves, from the neuropsychological point of view, psychological operations of reconfiguration of attentional processes, corporal consciousness, and cognitive reappraisal of reality [46].

In the treatment of obesity, mindfulness techniques seem very effective in attenuating automatic eating present in many obese patients, as well as in improving reactions to cravings and impulsivity, in addition to regulating the relationship between negative emotions and emotional eating, resulting in better control of weight [47]. Although research findings on the effectiveness of mindfulness meditation on weight reduction are promising, there is still little evidence that such favorable results are long lasting [47]. A recent meta-analysis evaluated 19 studies on the impact of mindfulness on individuals trying to lose weight and found significant weight reduction in participants of mindfulness interventions in most of the included studies, cautioning, however, that methodological problems and the variability between studies weaken this evidence.

Psychodynamic Psychotherapy

Psychodynamic psychotherapies consider obesity as a psychosomatic phenomenon, in which an unconscious psychic conflict would be the origin of its main clinical and behavioral manifestations. Psychodynamic techniques closely resemble psychoanalysis insofar as they value the therapist–patient relationship as a therapeutic resource more than other psychotherapeutic techniques. Beutel et al. [48, 49] compared psychodynamic psychotherapy to behavioral psychotherapy in obese inpatients, concluding that, despite methodological differences, the two approaches were equally effective in improving eating behaviors, well-being, body image, and life-satisfaction both in short and in mid-term. The mechanisms through which these psychotherapies act in obese patients are, nevertheless, obscure, but it is possible that due to their longer durations, psychodynamic psychotherapies may strength more lasting behavioral changes in aspects of daily life, as well as favoring the struggle against weight regain [50].

Final Considerations

Psychotherapeutic treatment options for patients using BIB are still poorly studied; for this reason, techniques for which there are more evidences of efficacy for the treatment of obesity should be preferentially adopted in this population. In this context, to date, psychotherapies based on CBT, IPT, and Mindfulness [51] were the most studied, with several studies showing its effectiveness, particularly in patients presenting pathological eating behaviors. However, it is important to keep in mind that methodological limitations of many studies make it difficult to generalize the results. Obesity should be seen as a multidimensional phenomenon, where behavior is only one of its many variables, whose complexity increases the challenge imposed on whichever professionals involved in their understanding, treatment and prevention. Dysfunctional eating behaviors of those suffering from obesity, possibly their best-studied psychopathological issues, can be explained as trait-dependent or state-dependent conditions. This means that obesity *directly* causes behavioral deviations, through several neurophysiopathological mechanisms, such as low-grade systemic inflammation, insulin resistance, and changes in the intestinal microbiome (state-dependent) processes that can affect the brain, damaging neurotransmission systems regulating mood, impulsiveness, and behavior. Such processes can be reversed with weight loss, as shown by some studies on the effects of bariatric surgery on the central nervous system [52]. However, trait-dependent conditions such as temperament, personality, and individual coping styles lie behind the various ways obesity *indirectly* alters an individual's behavior. Thus, certain temperamental characteristics may increase the odds of dysfunctional eating behaviors in obesity [53], defining, likewise, the chances of therapeutic success. For instance, conscientious and self-controlled individuals may adhere better to BIB treatment routines; otherwise, neurotic, impulsive and reward-sensible individuals, personality traits related to increased risk of weight gain [53], have higher chances of unfavorable outcomes. Further studies on psychological treatment for BIB users need to be performed, for example, to clarify which psychotherapeutic techniques are most effective and safe, both on short- and long-term, as well as whether they are best done when performed individually or in group.

References

1. Monsey MS, Gerhard DM. Obesity introduction. Yale J Biol Med. 2014;87(2):97–8.
2. Fernandes M, Atallah AN, Soares BG, Humberto S, Guimarães S, Matos D, Monteiro L, Richter B. Intragastric balloon for obesity. Cochrane Database Syst Rev. 2007 Jan 24;(1):CD004931. Review. PubMed PMID: 17253531.
3. Farina MG, Baratta R, Nigro A, Vinciguerra F, Puglisi C, Schembri R, et al. Intragastric balloon in association with lifestyle and/or pharmacotherapy in the long-term management of obesity. Obes Surg. 2012;22(4):565–71. https://doi.org/10.1007/s11695-011-0514-y.
4. Kotzampassi K, Grosomanidis V, Papakostas P, Penna S, Eleftheriadis E. 500 intragastric balloons: what happens 5 years thereafter? Obes Surg. 2012;22(6):896–903. https://doi.org/10.1007/s11695-012-0607-2.
5. Vranešić Bender D, Krznarić Z. Nutritional and behavioral modification therapies of obesity: facts and fiction. Dig Dis. 2012;30(2):163–7. https://doi.org/10.1159/000336670.
6. Teufel M, Becker S, Rieber N, Stephan K, Zipfel S. Psychotherapy and obesity: strategies challenges and possibilities. Nervenarzt. 2011;82(9):1133–9. https://doi.org/10.1007/s00115-010-3230-2.
7. Karasu SR. Psychotherapy-lite: obesity and the role of the mental health practitioner. Am J Psychother. 2013;67(1):3–22.
8. Cox AJ, West NP, Cripps AW. Obesity, inflammation, and the gut microbiota. Lancet Diabetes Endocrinol. 2015;3(3):207–15. https://doi.org/10.1016/S2213-8587(14)70134-2.
9. Miller AA, Spencer SJ. Obesity and neuroinflammation: a pathway to cognitive impairment. Brain Behav Immun. 2014;42:10–21. https://doi.org/10.1016/j.bbi.2014.04.001.
10. Zhao L. The gut microbiota and obesity: from correlation to causality. Nat Rev Microbiol. 2013;11(9):639–47. https://doi.org/10.1038/nrmicro3089.
11. Kullmann S, Heni M, Hallschmid M, Fritsche A, Preissl H, Häring HU. Brain insulin resistance at the crossroads of metabolic and cognitive disorders in humans. Physiol Rev. 2016;96(4):1169–209. https://doi.org/10.1152/physrev.00032.2015.
12. Berkowitz RI, Fabricatore AN. Obesity, psychiatric status, and psychiatric medications. Psychiatr Clin North Am. 2011;34(4):747–64. https://doi.org/10.1016/j.psc.2011.08.007.
13. Van Dorsten B, Lindley EM. Cognitive and behavioral approaches in the treatment of obesity. Med Clin North Am. 2011;95(5):971–88. https://doi.org/10.1016/j.mcna.2011.06.008.
14. Majanovic SK, Ruzic A, Bulian AP, Licul V, Orlic ZC, Stimac D. Comparative Study of Intragastric balloon and cognitive-behavioral approach for non-morbid obesity. Hepato-Gastroenterology. 2014;61(132):937–41.
15. Takihata M, Nakamura A, Aoki K, Kimura M, Sekino Y, Inamori M, et al. Comparison of intragastric balloon therapy and intensive lifestyle modification therapy with respect to weight reduction and abdominal fat distribution in super-obese Japanese patients. Obes Res Clin Pract. 2014;8(4):e331–8. https://doi.org/10.1016/j.orcp.2013.07.002.
16. Odom J, Zalesin KC, Washington TL, Miller WW, Hakmeh B, Zaremba DL, et al. Behavioral predictors of weight regain after bariatric surgery. Obes Surg. 2010;20(3):349–56. https://doi.org/10.1007/s11695-009-9895-6.
17. Peterson ND, Middleton KR, Nackers LM, Medina KE, Milsom VA, Perri MG. Dietary self-monitoring and long-term success with weight management. Obesity (Silver Spring). 2014;22(9):1962–7. https://doi.org/10.1002/oby.20807.

18. Burke LE, Wang J, Sevick MA. Self-monitoring in weight loss: a systematic review of the literature. J Am Diet Assoc. 2011;111(1):92–102. https://doi.org/10.1016/j.jada.2010.10.008.
19. Pearson ES. Goal setting as a health behavior change strategy in overweight and obese adults: a systematic literature review examining intervention components. Patient Educ Couns. 2012;87(1):32–42. https://doi.org/10.1016/j.pec.2011.07.018.
20. Michael RB, Garry M, Kirsch I. Suggestion, cognition, and behavior. Curr Dir Psychol Sci. 2012;21:151–6.
21. Miller CK, Bauman J. Goal setting: an integral component of effective diabetes care. Curr Diab Rep. 2014;14(8):509. https://doi.org/10.1007/s11892-014-0509-x.
22. Walker AK, Ibia IE, Zigman JM. Disruption of Cue-potentiated feeding in mice with blocked ghrelin signaling. Physiol Behav. 2012;108:34–43. https://doi.org/10.1016/j.physbeh.2012.10.003.
23. Volkow ND, Wang GJ, Fowler JS, Telang F. Overlapping neuronal circuits in addiction and obesity: evidence of systems pathology. Philos Trans R Soc Lond B Biol Sci. 2008;363(1507):3191–200. https://doi.org/10.1098/rstb.2008.0107.
24. Volkow ND, Wang GJ, Baler RD. Reward, dopamine and the control of food intake: implications for obesity. Trends Cogn Sci. 2011;15(1):37–46.
25. Carnell S, Gibson C, Benson L, Ochner CN, Geliebter A. Neuroimaging and obesity: current knowledge and future directions. Obes Rev. 2012;13(1):43–56.
26. Doolan KJ, Breslin G, Hanna D, Gallagher AM. Attentional bias to food-related visual cues: is there a role in obesity? Proc Nutr Soc. 2015;74(1):37–45. https://doi.org/10.1017/S002966511400144X.
27. Johnson AW. Eating beyond metabolic need: how environmental cues influence feeding behavior. Trends Neurosci. 2013;36(2):101–9. https://doi.org/10.1016/j.tins.2013.01.002.
28. Pagoto S, Appelhans BM. The challenge of stimulus control: a comment on Poelman et al. Ann Behav Med. 2015;49(1):3–4. https://doi.org/10.1007/s12160-014-9661-4.
29. Caudek C. Individual differences in cognitive control on self-referenced and other-referenced memory. Conscious Cogn. 2014;30:169–83. https://doi.org/10.1016/j.concog.2014.08.017.
30. Brown TG, Ouimet MC, Eldeb M, Tremblay J, Vingilis E, Nadeau L, et al. Personality, executive control, and neurobiological characteristics associated with different forms of risky driving. PLoS One. 2016;11(2):e0150227. https://doi.org/10.1371/journal.pone.0150227.
31. Murawski ME, Milsom VA, Ross KM, Rickel KA, DeBraganza N, Gibbons LM, et al. Problem solving, treatment adherence, and weight-loss outcome among women participating in lifestyle treatment for obesity. Eat Behav. 2009;10(3):146–51. https://doi.org/10.1016/j.eatbeh.2009.03.005.
32. Pierce D. Problem solving therapy – use and effectiveness in general practice. Aust Fam Physician. 2012;41(9):676–9.
33. Pierce D, Gunn J. Using problem solving therapy in general practice. Aust Fam Physician. 2007;36(4):230–3.
34. Hebebrand J, Albayrak Ö, Adan R, Antel J, Dieguez C, de Jong J, et al. "Eating addiction", rather than "food addiction", better captures addictive-like eating behavior. Neurosci Biobehav Rev. 2014;47:295–306. https://doi.org/10.1016/j.neubiorev.2014.08.016.
35. Stice E, Dieting PK. Eating disorders. In: Agras WS, editor. The Oxford handbook of eating disorders. New York: Oxford University Press; 2010. p. 148–78.
36. Volkow ND, Wang GJ, Tomasi D, Baler RD. The addictive dimensionality of obesity. Biol Psychiatry. 2013;73(9):811–8. https://doi.org/10.1016/j.biopsych.2012.12.020.
37. Melemis SM. Relapse prevention and the five rules of recovery. Yale J Biol Med. 2015;88(3):325–32.
38. Conceição EM, Mitchell JE, Engel SG, Machado PP, Lancaster K, Wonderlich SA. What is "grazing"? Reviewing its definition, frequency, clinical characteristics, and impact on bariatric surgery outcomes, and proposing a standardized definition. Surg Obes Relat Dis. 2014;10(5):973–82. https://doi.org/10.1016/j.soard.2014.05.002.
39. Corlett PR, Taylor JR, Wang XJ, Fletcher PC, Krystal JH. Toward a neurobiology of delusions. Prog Neurobiol. 2010;92:345–69.

40. Kringelbach ML, Berridge KC. The neurobiology of pleasure and happiness. In: Illes J, Sahakian BJ, editors. The Oxford handbook of neuroethics. Oxford: Oxford University Press; 2011. p. 15–32.
41. Lipsitz JD, Markowitz JC. Mechanisms of change in interpersonal therapy (IPT). Clin Psychol Rev. 2013;33(8):1134–47. https://doi.org/10.1016/j.cpr.2013.09.002.
42. Tanofsky-Kraff M, Wilfley DE, Young JF, Mufson L, Yanovski SZ, Glasofer DR, et al. A pilot study of interpersonal psychotherapy for preventing excess weight gain in adolescent girls at-risk for obesity. Int J Eat Disord. 2010;43(8):701–6. https://doi.org/10.1002/eat.20773.
43. Wilfley DE, Welch RR, Stein RI, Spurrell EB, Cohen LR, Saelens BE, et al. A randomized comparison of group cognitive behavioral therapy and group interpersonal psychotherapy for the treatment of overweight individuals with binge-eating disorder. Arch Gen Psychiatry. 2002;59(8):713–21.
44. Shomaker LB, Tanofsky-Kraff M, Matherne CE, Mehari RD, Olsen CH, Marwitz SE, et al. A randomized, comparative pilot trial of family-based interpersonal psychotherapy for reducing psychosocial symptoms, disordered-eating, and excess weight gain in at-risk preadolescents with loss-of-control-eating. Int J Eat Disord. 2017;50(9):1084–94. https://doi.org/10.1002/eat.22741.
45. Tonelli H. Cognição social, modo default e psicopatologia. Revista PsicoFAE: Pluralidades em Saúde Mental. 2016;4(1):19–32.
46. Grecucci A, Pappaianni E, Siugzdaite R, Theuninck A, Job R. Mindful emotion regulation: exploring the neurocognitive mechanisms behind mindfulness. Biomed Res Int. 2015;2015:1. https://doi.org/10.1155/2015/670724.
47. Mantzios M, Wilson JC. Mindfulness, eating behaviours, and obesity: a review and reflection on current findings. Curr Obes Rep. 2015;4(1):141–6. https://doi.org/10.1007/s13679-014-0131-x.
48. Beutel M, Thiede R, Wiltink J, Sobez I. Effectiveness of behavioral and psychodynamic inpatient treatment of severe obesity–first results from a randomized study. Int J Obes Relat Metab Disord. 2001;25(Suppl 1):96–8.
49. Beutel ME, Dippel A, Szczepanski M, Thiede R, Wiltink J. Mid-term effectiveness of behavioral and psychodynamic inpatient treatments of severe obesity based on a randomized study. Psychother Psychosom. 2006;75(6):337–45.
50. Becker S, Rapps N, Zipfel S. Psychotherapy in obesity: a systematic review. Psychother Psychosom Med Psychol. 2007;57(11):420–7.
51. Olson KL, Emery CF. Mindfulness and weight loss: a systematic review. Psychosom Med. 2015;77(1):59–67. https://doi.org/10.1097/PSY.0000000000000127.
52. Tonelli H, Sartori FM, Marchesini JCD, Marchesini JB, Tonelli D. Effects of bariatric surgery on the central nervous system and eating behavior in humans: a systematic review on the neuroimaging studies. J Bras Psiquiatr. 2013;62(4):297–305. https://doi.org/10.1590/S0047-20852013000400007.
53. Gerlach G, Herpertz S, Loeber S. Personality traits and obesity: a systematic review. Obes Rev. 2015;16(1):32–63. https://doi.org/10.1111/obr.12235.

Physical Activities

33

Anna Carolina Hoff and Sérgio Alexandre Barrichelo Júnior

Introduction

According to the World Health Organization, in 2010 there were over 1 billion overweight adults worldwide, with 400 million obese. This is a growing number that represents a health problem, even considered an epidemic on a global scale [9]. Obesity is a complex metabolic disease related to numerous comorbidities. In addition to physical harm, it also leads to psychological issues such as depression [4, 14].

The main cause of obesity is an imbalance between calories consumed and calories expenditure, thus generating an excessive amount of fat in the body. Its treatment can take different paths, mainly representing a change in life style that is meant to last for the entire individual's life. This change starts with dietary intervention, in some cases associated with physical exercises. However, this is not always effective, making other interventions necessary, such as pharmacological, surgical and minimally invasive techniques, such as the intragastric balloon (IGB) implant, subject of this book [4, 9].

Endoscopic bariatric therapy provides good efficacy with lower risks than conventional surgical procedures. Among the various endoscopic treatments for obesity, the intragastric balloon is associated with significant efficacy in body weight reduction and relief of comorbidities [11].

Even though surgery has a high probability of success, only true change in lifestyle, including the insertion of healthy habits, can lead to success in reaching ideal weight. During the IGB treatment, there is a gap of 4, 6, or 12 months (according to

A. C. Hoff (✉)
Department of Bariatric Endoscopy, Angioskope SP Endoscopic Center, São Paulo, SP, Brazil

S. A. Barrichelo Júnior
Department of Bariatric Endoscopy, Healthme Clinic, São Paulo, SP, Brazil
e-mail: sergio.barrichello@healthme.com.br

© Springer Nature Switzerland AG 2020
M. Galvao Neto et al. (eds.), *Intragastric Balloon for Weight Management*,
https://doi.org/10.1007/978-3-030-27897-7_33

the device chosen) to engage into these habit modifications. It is a small amount of time to develop consciousness on the importance of making the right dietary choices and the need to incorporate the practice of exercises [15].

Thus, this chapter aims to introduce the impact and risks of the practice of physical activity during IGB treatment.

Physical Activity and the Bariatric Patient

Prescription of exercises may sound like a simple and obvious solution to the bariatric patient, but physicians must be aware of both physical and psychological issues that involve engaging in such an activity. Sixty-five percent of obese patients complain of articulation pain, and even the lightest stimulation of knees and ankles can lead to discomfort and movement limitation. Impacts must be avoided at an early stage, at least until 10% of total body weight has been lost, in order to prevent inflammation or worsening of a previous condition. Shortness of breath is also an issue, due to the sedentary behavior itself, or because of the direct compression of the chest and abdomen by its increased volume, restraining proper inspiration [4, 15].

Adaptation to gym machines can be hard because most of them are ergonomic to a certain body weight that excludes obese patients, making them uncomfortable while using the equipment. If the physician or personal trainer cannot identify those difficulties, motivation and adherence to the training program will be low. Another concern is the psychological issues that involve prescribing and expecting the patient to follow a training routine. Most of IGB users are uncomfortable with their body shapes and do not have the courage to enroll at a gym and face a community that works out on a regular basis [4].

There is no doubt regarding the practice of physical activities and its benefits for the patient's life and health with regard not only for the maintenance of body mass. Patients that underwent IGB procedure follow the same logic of the ones that underwent bariatric surgery, however, with the gastric balloon patients are able to initiate physical activity earlier than surgical patients.

During the first week post IGB placement, there is an adaptation period when nausea, vomiting, and abdominal pain are very common. Symptoms control is a big challenge, and the correct medication support helps improve patient's quality of life, avoiding complaints and early IGB removal. As soon as the patient's condition starts to improve and these symptoms are no longer present, physical activity is recommended under supervision.

Bryner et al. [3] showed an important improvement in weight loss provided by physical activity associated to a very low-calorie diet (VLCD), in addition to an intensive, high volume resistance training program. This resulted in preservation of lean body weight (LBW) and resting metabolic rate (RMR) during weight loss with a VLCD [3].

The Benefits of Physical Activity

Physical activity may improve health in a wide range of ways, especially for obese patients. Regular activities are known to reduce the risk for cardiovascular diseases and type two diabetes by improving cardiac fitness, reducing blood pressure, and improving cellular sensibility to insulin. Additionally, it is good way of maintaining body weight after IGB placement [2, 17].

Beyond these advantages, an active lifestyle is greatly related to building a healthy and strong structure. This is related to the release of hormones that increase the body's ability to absorb amino acids and inhibit muscle breakdown [20].

Some psychological advantages of physical activities are also noteworthy. Exercise can play a role in the obese with depression, anxiety and stress, one of the main reasons that these patients have difficulty in adhering the regular workout as prescribed [7, 14]. Moreover, the brain suffers chemical changes, increasing its sensibility to serotonin and norepinephrine, modulating the symptoms of depression [1].

Deliopoulou et al. [6] demonstrated that signs of depression improved significantly in 40 patients, with some of those completely overcoming this comorbidity. Other metrics, such as BMI and body weight, also improved, and the quantity of subjects that were more depressed initially in the study also present a greater difference in body weight [6].

Sedentary lifestyle is one of the main causes of a great deal of diseases, such as obesity. One of the main obesity-related problems is metabolic syndrome, characterized by five major functional abnormalities: overweight, hypertension, insulin resistance, glucose intolerance, and dyslipidemia [8].

In a study by Speakman and Selman [19], the more an individual practiced physical activity, the higher his resting metabolic rate was, showing that the construction of healthy body mass, such as muscles, was responsible for this increase. An individual with a high resting metabolic rate spends more energy on a daily basis, making it is more difficult to return to a previous state of obesity [19].

To overcome some problems such as non-ergonomic equipment unfit for obese people, osteoarthritis, asthma, articular pain and depression, it is possible to apply the high-intensity interval training (HIIT) – also called sprint interval training. It is characterized by brief and intermittent bursts of activity alternated by rest periods of low intensity exercise. This sort of practice can be adapted to individualized goals. It is an interesting alternative to traditional exercises, leading to similar or even better psychological and physical results [10]. Even though it is not the best long-term approach to treat hyperlipidemia and obesity, or even improving muscle and bone mass, it's been proven to successfully reduce fat from the entire body [18].

Since there is no standard prescription for HIIT, it can be performed depending on the individual's resistance and can be done indoors, solving the problem with regard to the patient's will to leave home and practice exercise, whatever in a gym or outdoors. One may think doing exercises at home is not advisable, however, the patients may gain the necessary confidence to leave home and socialize. HIIT sections can take up to 30 minutes, meaning that for those who have little time for workout, it is a great option.

Obesity Treatment

The aim of physical activity prescription is to fulfill six major needs:

1. Potentialize weight loss.
2. Decrease body fat percentage.
3. Gain lean mass (muscular tissue) in order to increase the average metabolic rate.
4. Improve cardiovascular health.
5. Create a better self-image, promoting motivation on pursuing the weight target.
6. Socialize with people who share the same goals.

Normally the physical exercise program is prescribed as a 30 minute of moderate or intense activity, at least 5 days per week. Several aerobic exercises should be combined, so the individual does not become discontent, with better results than with practice of only one type of exercise. It is important to take into consideration each individual's limitations, since the obese patient may present some comorbidities that may influence exercise program choice [12].

Even though the practice of exercise may play an important role not only in improving weight but also in its maintenance, the prescription should take into consideration which programs to prescribe to those who underwent the IGB procedure, since they may represent different risks. Thus, Table 33.1 shows information regarding the physical activity its risk degree and consequence.

Some of these activities may cause discomfort during IGB treatment due to the excessive movement, causing motion of the balloon, consequently leading to nausea and vomiting. In addition to that, the risk is directly proportional to the chance of falling and having physical injuries that may harm the IGB device.

This takes us back to the practice of HIIT at home by depressive obese patients until they feel comfortable to get out and socialize. HIIT has a low risk of causing injuries, and even if it causes an accident, it has very low consequences and even lower probability to interfere with the IGB. Benefits from HIIT fulfill the patient's metabolic and psychological needs, with easy availability throughout the internet (either payed or free).

A study performed by Little et al. [13] compared HIIT with a continuous moderate-intensity exercise with regard to their impact on postprandial glycemic control on 10 inactive obese patients. The results for HIIT showed that a single session was able to improve postprandial glycemia during the next 24 hours, being superior than the continuous moderate-intensity exercise, once they presented a better result in the glucose levels after breakfast in the next day [13].

Racil et al. [16] evaluated the effect of HIIT and moderate-intensity interval training into maximal oxygen uptake, maximal aerobic speed, plasma lipids, and

Table 33.1 IGB risk table list of physical activities during obesity treatment

Training prescription	Risk	Consequence
Jogging	Very low	Medium
Walking	Very low	Very low
Bicycling	Low	Very low
Speed bicycling	High	High
Mountain bicycling	High	Very high
Skating	Medium	Medium
Roller skating	Medium	Medium
Swimmimg	Very low	Very low
Weightlifting	Very low	Very low
Diving	Very low	Medium
Baseball	Medium	Medium
Basketball	Medium	Medium
Roller hockey	Medium	Medium
Softball	Low	Low
Soccer	Low	Low
Tennis	Very low	Very low
Football	Low	Low
Rugby	High	Very high
Volleyball	Low	Low
Aerobic classes	Medium	Very low
Low impact aerobics	Very low	Very low
High impact aerobics	Medium	Very low
Step/Jump aerobic classes	Medium	Very low
Water aerobics	Medium	Very low
Ballet dancing	Very low	Very low
Zumba	Low	Very low
Judo	High	Very high
Jiu Jitsu	High	Very high
Karate	High	Very high
Tai-Kwon-Do	High	High
Boxing	Very low	Very high
Horse Riding	Very low	Very high
Polo	Very low	Very high
HIIT	Low	Very low

adiponectin levels of 34 obese adolescent females. All the metrics in the study groups changed positively, especially insulin resistance (HOMA-IR), showing an improvement of the metabolic syndrome that accompanies obesity. Only HIIT showed positive impact in waist circumference, triglyceride and total cholesterol levels [16].

The study from Dalzill et al. [5] evaluated intensive lifestyle intervention (HIIT and Mediterranean diet nutritional counselling) in relation to cardiometabolic and exercise parameters, in both metabolic healthy and unhealthy obese patients. Body mass, waist circumference, blood pressure, and insulin sensitivity were improved in both groups [5].

In addition to that, the improvement in resting metabolic index by the exercise itself means a greater muscle development, making it more difficult to get back to initial weigh. The higher this indicator, the bigger the chances that the patient has to overcome obesity and also maintain weight, which is a key part on the treatment, especially after undergoing a procedure such as a IGB placement [19].

Conclusion

Many physicians don't discuss physical activity with their patients because of time limitations or comfort-level constraints. This is unfortunate because the doctor's recommendations and proper guidance at the point of care are important predictors of patient participation in exercise.

References

1. Anderson E, Shivakumar G. Effects of exercise and physical activity on anxiety. Front Psych. 2013;4:27. https://doi.org/10.3389/fpsyt.2013.00027.
2. Booth FW, Roberts CK, Laye MJ. Lack of exercise is a major cause of chronic diseases. Compr Physiol. 2012;2(2):1143–211. https://doi.org/10.1002/cphy.c110025.
3. Bryner RW, Ullrich IH, Sauers J, Donley D, Hornsby G, Kolar M, Yeater R. Effects of resistance vs. aerobic training combined with an 800 calorie liquid diet on lean body mass and resting metabolic rate. J Am Coll Nutr. 1999;18(2):115–21.
4. Coen PM, Goodpaster BH. A role for exercise after bariatric surgery? Diabetes Obes Metab. 2016;18(1):16–23. https://doi.org/10.1111/dom.12545.
5. Dalzill C, Nigam A, Juneau M, Guilbeault V, Latour E, Mauriège P, Gayda M. Intensive lifestyle intervention improves cardiometabolic and exercise parameters in metabolically healthy obese and metabolically unhealthy obese individuals. Can J Cardiol. 2014;30(4):434–40. https://doi.org/10.1016/j.cjca.2013.11.033.
6. Deliopoulou K, Konsta A, Penna S, Papakostas P, Kotzampassi K. The impact of weight loss on depression status in obese individuals subjected to intragastric balloon treatment. Obes Surg. 2013;23(5):669–75. https://doi.org/10.1007/s11695-012-0855-1.
7. Ensari I, Sandroff BM, Motl RW. Effects of single bouts of walking exercise and yoga on acute mood symptoms in people with multiple sclerosis. Int J MS Care. 2016;18(1):1–8. https://doi.org/10.7224/1537-2073.2014-104.
8. Eriksson J, Taimela S, Koivisto VA. Exercise and the metabolic syndrome. Diabetologia. 1997;40(2):125–35. https://doi.org/10.1007/s001250050653.
9. Fock KM, Khoo J. Diet and exercise in management of obesity and overweight. J Gastroenterol Hepatol. 2013;28:59–63. https://doi.org/10.1111/jgh.12407.
10. Gibala MJ, Little JP, MacDonald MJ, Hawley JA. Physiological adaptations to low-volume, high-intensity interval training in health and disease. J Physiol. 2012;590(5):1077–84. https://doi.org/10.1113/jphysiol.2011.224725.
11. Kim SH, Chun HJ, Choi HS, Kim ES, Keum B, Jeen YT. Current status of intragastric balloon for obesity treatment. World J Gastroenterol. 2016;22(24):5495–504. https://doi.org/10.3748/wjg.v22.i24.5495.
12. Lecube A, Monereo S, Rubio MÁ, Martínez-de-Icaya P, Martí A, Salvador J, Masmiquel L, Goday A, Bellido D, Lurbe E, García-Almeida JM, Tinahones FJ, García-Luna PP, Palacio E, Gargallo M, Bretón I, Morales-Conde S, Caixàs A, Menéndez E, Puig-Domingo M, Casanueva FF. Prevention, diagnosis, and treatment of obesity. 2016 position statement of the Spanish Society for the Study of obesity. Endocrinol Diabetes y Nutrición (English ed). 2017;64:15–22. https://doi.org/10.1016/j.endien.2017.03.007.
13. Little JP, Jung ME, Wright AE, Wright W, Manders RJF. Effects of high-intensity interval exercise versus continuous moderate-intensity exercise on postprandial glycemic control assessed by continuous glucose monitoring in obese adults. Appl Physiol Nutr Metabol. 2014;39(7):835–41. https://doi.org/10.1139/apnm-2013-0512.
14. Livhits M, Mercado C, Yermilov I, Parikh JA, Dutson E, Mehran A, Ko CY, Gibbons MM. Exercise following bariatric surgery: systematic review. Obes Surg. 2010;20(5):657–65. https://doi.org/10.1007/s11695-010-0096-0.

15. Nisell R, Mizrah J. Knee and ankle joint forces during steps and jumps down from two different heights. Clin Biomech (Bristol, Avon). 1988;3(2):92–100. https://doi.org/10.1016/0268-0033(88)90051-4.
16. Racil G, Ben Ounis O, Hammouda O, Kallel A, Zouhal H, Chamari K, Amri M. Effects of high vs. moderate exercise intensity during interval training on lipids and adiponectin levels in obese young females. Eur J Appl Physiol. 2013;113(10):2531–40. https://doi.org/10.1007/s00421-013-2689-5.
17. Slentz CA, Houmard JA, Kraus WE. Exercise, abdominal obesity, skeletal muscle, and metabolic risk: evidence for a dose response. Obesity (Silver Spring). 2009;17(Suppl 3):S27–33. https://doi.org/10.1038/oby.2009.385.
18. Smith-Ryan AE, Melvin MN, Wingfield HL. High-intensity interval training: modulating interval duration in overweight/obese men. Phys Sportsmed. 2015;43(2):107–13. https://doi.org/10.1080/00913847.2015.1037231.
19. Speakman JR, Selman C. Physical activity and resting metabolic rate. Proc Nutr Soc. 2003;62(3):621–34. https://doi.org/10.1079/pns2003282.
20. Wolfe RR. Skeletal muscle protein metabolism and resistance exercise. J Nutr. 2006;136(2):525s–8s.

Index

© Springer Nature Switzerland AG 2020
M. Galvão Neto et al. (eds.), *Intragastric Balloon for Weight Management*,
https://doi.org/10.1007/978-3-030-27897-7

Printed in the United States
by Baker & Taylor Publisher Services